om

The Willingness to Pay
for Medical Care

The Willingness to Pay for Medical Care

Evidence from Two Developing Countries

Paul Gertler
Jacques van der Gaag

Published for the World Bank
The Johns Hopkins University Press
Baltimore and London

The Johns Hopkins University Press
Baltimore, Maryland 21211, U.S.A.

The findings, interpretations, and conclusions expressed in this book are those of the authors and do not necessarily represent the views and policies of the World Bank or its Board of Executive Directors or the countries they represent. The World Bank does not guarantee the accuracy of the data included in this publication and accepts no responsibility whatsoever for any consequences of their use.

Library of Congress Cataloging in Publication Data

Gertler, Paul, 1955–
   The willingness to pay for medical care : evidence from two
developing countries / Paul Gertler, Jacques van der Gaag.
     p. cm.
   Includes bibliographical references and index.
   ISBN 0-8018-4146-1
   1. Medical economics—Developing countries. 2. Medical care—
Developing countries—Finance. I. Gaag, J. van der. II. Title.
RA410.55.D48G47 1990
338.4′33621′091724—dc20   90-41549
                                   CIP

Contents

Acknowledgments

This study could not have been completed without the help and encouragement of many of our colleagues. We owe much to David de Ferranti, who suggested this study to us and whose early writings on the topic of health care financing are still influential in the debate. Avi Dor was instrumental in the design of the study and contributed significantly to the empirical results. Luis Locay and Warren Sanderson contributed key insights into the development of the empirical framework. Ruben Suarez-Berenguela provided the background information on Peru in his study (1988), upon which we draw freely and extensively in chapter 3. Excellent research and programming assistance were provided at various stages by Kalpana Mehra, Saad Shire, and Jorge Castillo.

We received critical and useful comments on earlier drafts from Bela Balassa, Jere Behrman, Nancy Birdsall, Angus Deaton, Dennis de Tray, Paul Glewwe, Margaret Grosh, Michael Grossman, Emmanuel Jimenez, William McGreevey, Phillip Musgrove, Germano Mwabu, Joseph Newhouse, John Newman, Mead Over, T. Paul Schultz, and anonymous referees. In all cases these led to significant improvements in the manuscript. Since we were selective in following the recommendations, we alone will be responsible for any mistakes or misinterpretations.

We would like to thank participants in the following seminars and conferences, who helped us to correct mistakes and clarify the exposition: seminars held at Erasmus University, Harvard University, Johns Hopkins University, State University of New York at Stony Brook, the University of Pennsylvania, the World Bank, and Yale University; and the meetings of the Population Association of America (Chicago, 1987), the European Econometric Society (Copenhagen, 1987, and Bologna, 1988), the Latin American Econometric Society (Costa Rica, 1988), and the North American Econometric Society (New York, 1988).

We are very grateful to Angela Murphy and Maria Paz Felix for typing and retyping the numerous drafts of the chapters. Brenda Rosa deserves gratitude for allowing us to draw on her editorial skills in putting it all together.

Guide to the Reader

Readers who want to get an overview of the contents of this book are advised to read chapter 1, the summary sections of chapters 2 through 7, and all of chapter 8. Those who want to familiarize themselves with the general issues of health care financing in developing countries should read chapter 2 and, for more detail on health care infrastructure, chapter 3. Those two chapters can be skipped by readers who are thoroughly familiar with health care systems in the developing world and their financing problems.

Chapter 4 is a nontechnical chapter introducing some concepts of welfare economics as they relate to health care. This chapter should help noneconomists follow the analysis presented in subsequent chapters.

Chapter 5 contains the main theoretical part of this study. It is rather technical, but it is a must for those readers who want to scrutinize the theoretical base of our empirical work. This work is presented in chapter 6, which is perhaps the most important.

Readers not interested in the details of the theoretical and empirical work could make do with reading only the summaries of chapters 5 and 6 and turning immediately to chapter 7, which covers the implications of our findings for policy. This chapter and the concluding one are recommended to anyone who took the trouble of picking up this book.

1
Introduction

This book is about money—money to pay for delivering health services in developing countries. The health status of the population in developing countries is well below that in industrial countries, and the distribution as well as the quality of health care in developing countries leave much to be desired. It is well known that the scarcity of resources for health care in developing countries is a primary cause of this state of affairs.

The first chapters of this book show the importance of health care in the development process. We speculate why governments, in both industrial and developing countries, are so involved in providing medical care, and we illustrate the shortcomings of the health care infrastructure in developing countries. Our account is based on detailed information from two countries, Côte d'Ivoire and Peru. These countries are used as case studies for the specific, relatively narrow question we attempt to answer: Are user fees for medical care a desirable and feasible alternative to government financing?

In many developing countries, governments provide most of the resources for the health care system. Subsidies for medical education, capital for government-run hospitals, subsidized drugs, and free services in clinics and hospitals are the rule, not the exception. In this respect, developing countries do not differ much from industrial countries in which the government's intervention in health care ranges from allotting subsidies for certain groups (such as the aged) through public health insurance to providing medical care free of charge to the entire population.

The main difference between health care in industrial and developing countries is that in the latter resources are much scarcer. Although there are many other problems—such as inefficient use of available resources, bias toward curative rather than preventive care, and preferential treatment of politically powerful constituencies—the lack of resources seems most pressing. This problem became worse during the global recession of the 1980s. Oil shocks in the 1970s and early 1980s, combined with tight monetary and fiscal policies in industrial countries, triggered this recession. Oil-importing developing countries were particularly hard hit, but many other countries suffered from low prices for their commodity exports and from low demand for their products. The developing world resorted to heavy borrowing, which, combined with the sharp increase in interest rates, skyrocketed the cost of debt service. For example, Cline (1983) reports that in 1973–77 15.4 percent of earnings from exports were used to service the debt. In 1985 many countries in Africa and Latin America spent 30 to 55 percent of their export earnings on debt service (see, for example, Kakwani 1988).

Faced with severe imbalances in their economies, developing countries started structural adjustment programs under the auspices of the International Monetary Fund and the World Bank. A typical adjustment package includes tight fiscal and monetary restraints and usually results in a significant fall in domestic output, real wages, and private consumption. Some observers, such as Cornia, Jolly, and Stewart (1987), have argued that austerity measures have put an unacceptable burden on the poor in these countries, especially through cuts in spending on social services such as food subsidies, health care, and education. Others, such as Behrman (1988) and Behrman and Deolalikar (1988a), assert that the evidence for adverse effects on the poor is mixed. Few, however, question the necessity of stabilization and adjustment measures for countries with unsustainable imbalances in their economies.

It is well beyond the scope of this book to discuss the pros and cons of the macroeconomic policies currently promoted by international development agencies. For our purposes, the relevance of the macroeconomic situation in developing countries lies in the recognition that resources are severely constrained, that a return to sustainable economic growth appears to take more time than initially expected, and that fiscal constraint profoundly affects the policies put in place to promote such growth.

This last point has an immediate bearing on our study. If the health care systems in developing countries suffer from lack of resources and if government expenditure is not likely to increase, what must be done to find the necessary resources to improve the health care structure? The common answers to this question are to use current resources more efficiently and to introduce (or increase) user fees; that is, let the consumer (the patient) pay a larger share of the cost. We shall focus on user fees in this book.

The feasibility and desirability of raising revenue from patients depend on the price sensitivity of the demand for medical care. There are three issues. First, how price elastic is the demand for medical care in general? Clearly, if small increases in the price greatly reduce utilization, the amount of extra revenue raised will be small, perhaps too small to justify the policy. Second, is the demand for medical care more or less price sensitive for some groups than for others? For instance, if the poor, the aged, women, or children are more price sensitive than, say, relatively well-to-do adult males, user fees may have consequences for the distribution of health care that are socially or politically undesirable. Finally, the desirability of expanding the utilization of medical care depends on the extent to which its use improves health. In this research we take as given the notion that medical care is efficacious. In some cases, however, quality is so low that this assumption could be suspect.

The main part of this study is devoted to answering the first two questions by analyzing the choice of health care provider made by households in rural communities in two developing countries. The answers to these questions are simple: yes, the demand for medical care is price sensitive, but not so much so that user fees cannot be a viable option for resource mobilization. And yes, the poor as well as children will be hurt more by the introduction of user fees than will the population in general.

These empirical results are presented in chapter 6. Their implications for policy are demonstrated in chapter 7, where we simulate the consequences of various pricing policies. These consequences are evaluated according to three criteria: the effect on the utilization of health care (including the distributional aspects), the potential for raising revenue, and the effect on the economic welfare of the population.

These two chapters form the core of the empirical study. The rest of the book is devoted to defining the problem and developing a theoretical framework for the analysis. In chapter 2 we illustrate the importance of health in the development process. In this chapter we also describe and evaluate the main arguments that are usually put forward to justify extensive government involvement in the health care system. Chapter 3 provides background information on health and medical care on two continents: Africa and South America, with emphasis on Côte d'Ivoire and Peru. Chapters 4 and 5 provide the analytical and theoretical underpinnings of our empirical work.

In the concluding chapter we rejoin the debate on user fees for medical care. We also discuss some of the caveats of our study and provide, among other things, an agenda for future research. In the final section of that chapter we give suggestions on how, armed with the new empirical evidence, government officials can introduce user fees for health care while also protecting the poor against the adverse effects of user fees.

2
Health, Health Care, and Development

In almost all countries, governments have been intervening in medical care markets. In this chapter we explain some of the reasons for this phenomenon and describe the various forms of intervention. How medical care is financed is only one part of the general questions of how medical markets perform and what their role is in health and development. Since we later analyze price responses, here we will highlight the role of financing in the political economy of medical care.

To place financing issues in context, we must understand why the health sector is so important to developing countries, why governments intervene in health care markets, how governments use additional financing, and what problems governments face in developing policies of intervention. This chapter is not meant to be a comprehensive treatment of these issues but rather an overview of the debate on financing health care in developing countries.

The health status of the population is one of the most important factors in the process of economic development for at least two reasons. First, as an indicator of economic development, it shows the success or failure of a country in providing for the most basic needs of its people (food, sanitary conditions, shelter, and so on). Second, health—a form of human capital—is a factor in the further development of a country. Health influences the supply and productivity of adults in the labor force and the enrollment and performance of children in school (Strauss 1986, Deolalikar 1988, Behrman and Deolalikar 1988b). Furthermore, high infant and child mortality rates greatly influence fertility rates, which, in turn, play a crucial role in development. (See, among others, Krueger 1968, World Bank 1980, Wheeler 1980, Hicks 1980, and Balassa 1985 for a discussion of the role of human capital in economic development.)

The correlation between crude health indicators, such as child mortality and life expectancy at birth, and per capita income is well documented (as, for example, in Preston 1980, Golladay and Liese

1980, World Bank 1980, and Caldwell 1986). So too is the correlation between expenditures for medical care and per capita income. Indeed, as we will show, this correlation is so strong that, especially in the case of poor countries, knowledge of a country's per capita income suffices to predict fairly accurately its per capita expenditures for medical goods and services.

Given that the goal of medical care is to improve the health status of the population and given the correlation between health and economic development and between development and health care expenditures, one might expect a somewhat stronger relation between health status and medical care expenditures than is usually found. In examining this issue, our aim is not to develop a model that shows the causal relations among the three variables of health, health care, and development. Rather, by showing the correlations, we want to highlight some reasons that the health status of a population is of primary concern to policymakers in the developing world as well as in industrial countries. This concern is frequently manifested in heavy government involvement in the health care sector, ranging from the provision of public health insurance for selected groups to the constitutional right of every citizen to have access to free medical care.

Next we discuss other issues that help explain why in most countries the government is very involved in providing medical care. Although in many respects health care is a normal good, with positive income and negative price elasticities, certain aspects of health and medical care make it less desirable to let market forces alone regulate the provision of medical goods and services. This does not necessarily mean that government intervention is a panacea. But it does help to explain the involvement of governments in health care.

In the last section of this chapter we turn to the merits and potential hazards of government intervention in the market for medical goods and services. We discuss in general terms the various forms of intervention, especially as they relate to the financing of health care. We also acknowledge the financial and structural constraints that governments face. After presenting a simple descriptive analysis based on aggregate data from thirty-four countries for the year 1975, we present the background for chapter 3's more detailed and country-specific discussion of how two health care markets are organized and financed.

Health and Development

There is a strong positive correlation between health and development. This is demonstrated in figure 2–1, in which four health indicators—life expectancy at birth, infant and child mortality rates, and crude death rate—are plotted against gross national product (GNP) per capita. The countries chosen are the same as those included in Kravis, Heston, and Summers (1982) and represent all stages of development.[1] The countries are listed in table 2–1 in ascending order of GNP per capita. (Double logarithmic regressions for the sample are presented in table 2–2.)

These familiar diagrams demonstrate the wide variation of health status across countries. Life expectancy at birth ranges from 41.7 years in Malawi to 74.6 years in the Netherlands. Infant mortality rates range from 10.3 per thousand live births to 184.0 per thousand, and the crude death rate ranges from 6.2 per thousand people to 23.3 per thousand.

The diagrams also show the very strong correlation between health status and income levels. The associated regression coefficients in

Figure 2-1. Health Indicators and GNP per Capita for Selected Countries, 1975
(logarithm)

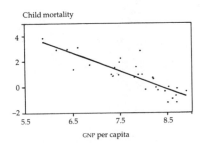

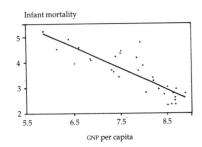

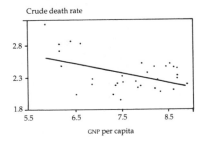

Note: The lines drawn through the scatter diagrams represent double logarithmic regressions. See table 2-1 for a list of the countries represented.
Source: World Bank 1986.

table 2–2 are all significantly different from zero at a confidence level of better than 1 percent, and the adjusted R^2 values show that per capita income is a fairly good predictor of health status except in the case of the crude death rate. The regression results suggest that a 10 percent increase in GNP per capita corresponds roughly with a one-year increase in life expectancy at birth, an 8.3 percent reduction in

Table 2-1. GNP per Capita for Selected Countries, 1975
(1975 U.S. dollars)

Country	GNP per capita
Malawi	351
Kenya	470
India	470
Pakistan	590
Sri Lanka	667
Zambia	737
Thailand	936
Philippines	996
Korea, Rep.	1,484
Malaysia	1,540
Colombia	1,608
Jamaica	1,722
Syrian Arab Rep.	1,794
Brazil	1,811
Romania	2,386
Mexico	2,487
Yugoslavia	2,591
Iran, Islamic Rep.	2,704
Uruguay	2,844
Ireland	3,048
Hungary	3,558
Poland	3,597
Italy	3,861
Spain	4,010
United Kingdom	4,587
Japan	4,906
Austria	4,994
Netherlands	5,397
Belgium	5,574
France	5,876
Luxembourg	5,883
Denmark	5,910
Germany	5,952
United States	7,176

Source: Kravis, Heston, and Summers 1982.

the infant mortality rate, a 14.2 percent reduction in the child mortality rate, and a 1.5 percent reduction in the crude death rate.

Development and the Consumption of Health Care

Income alone does not produce good health. There is ample evidence, from both microeconomic and macroeconomic studies, that income is a proxy for improved nutritional status, more sanitary conditions, better housing, higher levels of education, and so on (Preston 1980). All of these factors contribute directly or indirectly to an improvement in overall health status. The most direct way of improving health, however, is to provide medical goods and services.

Figure 2–2 shows the relation between per capita expenditures on health care and GNP per capita. Per capita expenditures in this sample of countries range from $8.70 in Kenya to $401.29 in the United States. The double logarithmic Engel curve drawn through the scatter diagram has an adjusted R^2 of 0.940 and indicates that medical care is a luxury good: the income elasticity of total health care expenditures is 1.329 (table 2–3). This finding is not new. Musgrove (1978) reports income elasticities ranging from about 0.81 to 1.34, using data on household income and expenditure from ten South American cities. In a later study (1983), Musgrove again concludes that health care is a luxury good (that is, that income elasticity exceeds 1.0). Newhouse (1977), using a data set similar to ours but for industrial countries only, obtained income elasticities in the range of 1.13 to 1.31. The persistently high correlation between health care expenditures and per capita income shows that despite numerous efforts to keep health care costs down, as evidenced by the large variety of health care systems, insurance schemes, and other financing mechanisms in existence, in

Table 2-2. Health Indicators and Economic Development for Selected Countries

Item	Life expectancy at birth	Infant mortality	Child mortality	Crude death rate
Constant	2.951	10.024	11.851	3.510
	(26.84)	(14.96)	(11.52)	(8.75)
GNP per capita	0.157	−0.833	−1.415	−0.151
	(11.09)	(9.65)	(10.68)	(2.91)
$\bar{R}^2$	0.787	0.737	0.774	0.185

Note: Coefficients are estimated from double logarithmic regressions (*T* values in parentheses). See table 2-1 for a list of the countries represented.

Figure 2-2. Health Care Expenditures and GNP per Capita for Selected Countries
(logarithm)

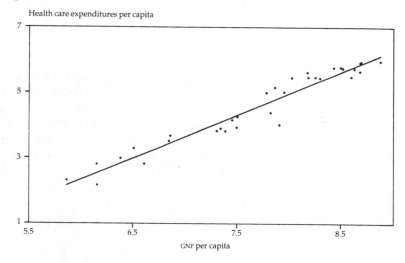

Note: See table 2-1 for a list of the countries represented.
Source: Data from Kravis, Heston, and Summers 1982.

the end countries consume an amount of medical care that is determined mainly by their level of income.

This conclusion foreshadows one of the main issues dealt with in this book: how to maintain and, indeed, improve a health care system in the light of constant or contracting resources. As we argue later, many developing countries face declining GNPs per capita, increasing demand for medical care, worsening budgetary problems, and contracting private consumption. Furthermore, their health care systems already leave much to be desired: hospitals without equipment, doctors without drugs, and rural clinics without safe drinking water or electricity are often the rule rather than the exception. In periods of sustained economic growth, the health care system might be expected to show more than a proportional improvement (at least with regard to expenditures), given the apparently high income elasticity of medical care. By the same token, it would seem that special attention needs to be given to the health care system in times of economic recession or zero economic growth (see World Health Organization 1987a and 1987b). Where are the resources to maintain the current system? How can additional resources be generated to make the necessary improvements? These questions are central to this study.

Table 2-3. Average Health Care Expenditure per Capita and Regression Results of Health Care Expenditure on GNP
(logarithm)

Item	Per capita expenditure			Regression result			
	Average	Standard error	Share of total (percent)	Constant		Income elasticity		$\overline{R}^2$
Drugs and medical preparations	34.74	45.08	20.7	−6.791	(7.74)	1.276	(11.29)	0.793
Medical supplies	4.27	10.34	2.5	−4.924	(2.72)	0.691	(2.97)	0.191
Therapeutic equipment	4.81	7.19	2.9	−11.798	(5.48)	1.613	(5.81)	0.499
Physicians' services	37.64	49.17	22.4	−9.618	(11.26)	1.627	(14.79)	0.868
Dental services	9.25	13.36	5.5	−17.564	(11.29)	2.409	(12.02)	0.813
Nursing services	28.27	39.23	16.8	−9.048	(10.17)	1.519	(13.20)	0.840
Hospital care	49.25	65.73	29.3	−7.272	(6.61)	1.361	(9.61)	0.735
Total	168.23	215.81	100.0	−5.640	(12.45)	1.329	(22.77)	0.940

Note: Figures in parentheses are T values. Data from Kravis, Heston, and Summers 1982.

Table 2–3 shows summary statistics and Engel curves (in logarithmic form) for detailed per capita expenditures on health care. Hospitals and physicians' services are the largest categories of expenditure, but drugs and nurses also command large shares of the total health care budget. With the exception of medical supplies, all items are luxuries in the economic sense: for the luxury items, income elasticities range from 1.361 for hospitals to 2.409 for dental services. The overall income elasticity is 1.329. The variation in elasticities implies that the shares within the health care budget will change as a country develops. We show this in figure 2–3 for an average country.

Health Production Functions

Although income is a good predictor of a nation's health status as measured by such crude indicators as mortality rates and life expectancy, at the microeconomic level many complex factors influence individual health status. A health production function aggregated over all individuals could summarize the complex causal chains that affect individual health. We will estimate the simplest such aggregated reduced-form health production function. The nature of the data available prevents the formulation of a convincing structural

Figure 2-3. Breakdown of Health Care Budget and GNP per Capita

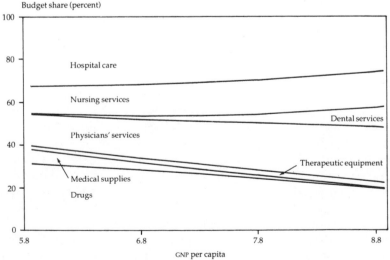

Source: Data from Kravis, Heston, and Summers 1982.

model that shows how governments, by using their scarce resources rationally, are able to improve the health of their population and how, in turn, this improved health contributes to economic development. Our goal is much less pretentious and is in the same spirit as the descriptive analyses in the preceding two sections. We want to investigate whether the more than proportional increase in health care expenditures that accompanies economic growth contributes to improving the health of the population.

Factors other than medical care, however, are relevant to a population's health status; these include education, overall consumption levels, and general living conditions. As a proxy measure for education we use the illiteracy rate. We expect individual and household consumption levels to be important, especially with regard to food consumption. Average calorie intake is used as a proxy for food consumption. Overall living conditions may be assessed by examining access to public services, safe drinking water, safe sewerage systems, and so on. Although it is far from being an ideal measure, we will use population density as a proxy for overall living conditions. The health measures used are the same as those introduced in the preceding section, and the consumption of medical goods and services is represented by per capita health care expenditures. The health production functions are estimated in double logarithmic form.

Estimation results are presented in table 2–4. The results should be interpreted with caution given the obvious problems of simultaneity. The results, however, are similar to those obtained by Rao (1989), who attempts to control for simultaneity.

Perhaps the most surprising result of this simple exercise is that literacy stands out as a very important factor in the production of health. Many studies based on microeconomic data have shown that parents' education, for example, is an important determinant of children's health status (Strauss 1987, for example). Others (such as Behrman and Wolfe 1987, Wolfe and Behrman 1984 and 1987, Barrera 1987 and 1990, and Thomas, Strauss, and Henriques 1987) showed that the link between education and health weakens when unobserved family background characteristics are controlled. Evidence from aggregated data is more scarce, but Cochrane, O'Hara, and Leslie (1980) also report strong correlations between adult literacy and measures of children's health.

If population density is an appropriate proxy for overall living conditions, the results show that infant and child mortality rates fall when these conditions improve. Calorie intake does not show any significant effect on health. Most likely, the distribution of food consumption, as, for example, calories consumed by the poorest 20 percent of the population, is more relevant to health than the average calorie intake (see, for instance, Behrman and Deolalikar 1987). The use of national averages obscures the relation between health and nutritional status that has been demonstrated in studies using microeconomic data.

The most important result of the estimation is the correlation of health care expenditures with health. The estimation results indicate that a 10 percent increase in health care expenditures is associated with an increase of 0.4 years in life expectancy at birth, a 4.1 percent reduction in the infant mortality rate (from 50.7 to 48.6 per thousand on average), and an 8.7 percent reduction in the child mortality rate (from 6.35 to 5.80 per thousand). A 10 percent increase in expenditures corresponds to $1.00 per capita for the poorest country in this sample and to $16.82 per capita on average. Health and medical care move procyclically. Just as sustained economic growth can be expected to lead to improved health, other things being equal, so a decline in per capita income is likely to result in a deterioration of the health care system and a subsequent reduction in health status.[2]

Despite the plausibility of these results, we caution the reader not to take these estimates as proof that under all circumstances an increase or decrease in health care expenditures will result in an improvement in or reduction of the population's health status. The causal chain that produces good health is a complex one that cannot

Table 2-4. Health Production Functions
(logarithm)

Item	Life expectancy at birth	Infant mortality	Child mortality	Crude death rate
Constant	3.110	10.251	4.752	0.454
	(5.22)	(1.80)	(0.57)	(0.15)
Literacy	0.191	−0.400	−0.708	−0.658
	(7.06)	(1.54)	(1.88)	(4.84)
Population density	0.009	−0.169	−0.238	−0.007
	(1.38)	(2.54)	(2.46)	(0.19)
Calorie intake	−0.013	−0.289	0.538	0.608
	(0.16)	(0.38)	(0.49)	(1.54)
Health care expenditures per capita	0.062	−0.412	−0.868	−0.014
	(3.56)	(2.48)	(3.60)	(0.16)
$\bar{R}^2$	0.941	0.819	0.862	0.571

Note: Figures in parentheses are *T* values. Data are from World Bank 1986.

be adequately analyzed using aggregated data. Nonetheless, although health care expenditures can be wasteful or even counterproductive, there is, in general, a direct causal relation between health care consumption and improved health. Moreover, our results correspond to those based on studies, using mostly microeconomic data, that attempt to show the causal relations between income, education, and the use of health services on the one hand and improved health on the other (Rosenzweig and Schultz 1982 and 1983 and Rosenzweig and Wolpin 1986, for example).

Government Intervention in the Health Care Sector

The relations among health, health care utilization, and development explain, at least in part, the political will of many governments to increase the consumption of medical care, as through subsidies or by providing health care free of charge. Increased consumption of medical care would be expected to reduce suffering and increase health status (and, by extension, productivity). Thus there is strong justification for government intervention in the market for medical goods and services. Our results are consistent with the claim that such government efforts result in a healthier population.

There are many other good reasons for governments to intervene in the provision of certain types of medical care. Not all forms of medical care, however, are equally effective in improving the overall health of the population. Furthermore, most kinds of market intervention come at a cost, be it in the form of reduced efficiency or, when the price mechanism is being replaced by some other form of rationing, in the form of undesirable inequity. Finally, and perhaps most important, governments face budgetary constraints. Without due respect for such constraints, even the best intentions of governments are doomed to fail. It is often argued that the neglect of budgetary realities, combined with other negative side effects of government intervention in the health care market, accounts for the dismal state of many health care systems in the developing world.

Still, as already stated, there are several good reasons for the provision of medical goods and services not to be left to market forces alone. First, it is well recognized that the consumption of medical care can generate externalities. Health care programs that generate large externalities include vaccination programs, sanitation programs, the provision of clean drinking water, and medical research. Though not all externalities necessarily call for government intervention, some aspects of medical care, such as the control of contagious diseases, are best provided by the government.

Second, spells of bad health are uncertain events, which makes the need to spend on medical care unpredictable. Arrow, in a seminal article (1963), stressed the unpredictability of medical outlays, thus providing the formal argument for the economic (welfare-enhancing) efficiency of implementing some form of health insurance. Often such insurance is provided by the government, either in the form of comprehensive public insurance schemes or by providing medical care at subsidized prices or free of charge.

Finally, and perhaps more important than all other arguments combined, good health is widely perceived as a basic human right. Financial or other barriers to obtaining medical care are thought to be unethical or at least socially undesirable. This belief has in some countries resulted in the constitutional right of all citizens to obtain medical care free of charge. In other countries governments have taken the role of the sole provider of medical care, usually with accompanying public insurance schemes. The belief that health is a basic human right also underlies the declaration of Alma Ata, which aims at "Health for All" by the year 2000.

Whatever the motives of government intervention in the health care market, the policies established under such intervention result in a reduction in what the consumer pays for medical care. This price reduction, in turn, has led to two widespread phenomena that have given rise to more government intervention: moral hazard and supplier-induced demand. Since any type of insurance lowers the price of the insured good to the consumer, at least at the time that the transaction takes place, the consumer has an incentive to buy more of the good than he or she otherwise would (if the good is price elastic). This phenomenon is referred to in the insurance literature as a moral hazard and is sometimes said to contribute to the alleged overutilization of some kinds of medical care. Regulations to counter this undesirable side effect of health insurance include requiring consultations with general practitioners before obtaining more expensive care from specialists or hospitals, as well as establishing deductibles and copayments.

The term supplier-induced demand refers to the possibility that physicians may, in part, pursue their own interests when prescribing treatment. Since the fully insured patient has no incentive to search for the most cost-effective treatment, and indeed may perceive the most expensive treatment as the best one, the physician may prescribe and deliver the treatment that is most profitable. The literature on supplier-induced demand is quite extensive though far from conclusive (see, for example, Phelps 1986). Measures to reduce the demand-increasing effects include compulsory second opinions for major operations and innovative insurance schemes that offer incentives for the physician to search for more cost-effective treatments (see the extensive literature on health maintenance organizations, such as Welch 1985).

The hypothesis of supplier-induced demand depends on the supposed ignorance of consumers in the health care market. The patient suffering from a disease knows that he or she needs some form of medical care but usually does not know what kind and quantity of drug or treatment is needed. This situation has led to a wide range of regulatory measures to protect the consumer. Health care workers need to fulfill minimum requirements to obtain a license to practice, and medical education is generally provided by the government or strongly regulated. Drugs can be marketed only after extensive testing, and many drugs can be provided only by licensed pharmacists.

Three Categories of Health Care

Many special aspects of health and medical care provide compelling reasons for some government intervention in the health care market. Indeed, the health care system is among the most regulated industries in the world. All interventions will, directly or indirectly, alter the price of the good or service to the consumer. For instance, restrictions on entering the market, such as licensing, are likely to raise the price of medical care. Most other interventions, however, are meant to reduce the price, through direct subsidies, public health insurance, or, in some cases, the public provision of free medical care.

These price reductions will, in principle, increase the consumption of medical care and, consequently, improve the health status of the population. Given the importance of health as a public good and as an important factor in development, this seems a good thing, but it is important to realize that health care is not a homogeneous commodity. It includes drugs, physicians' services, hospital and nursing home care, immunization campaigns, sanitation services, and health education programs on such topics as the benefits of regular exercise, the hazards of smoking, and the importance of preparing food in a sanitary way and boiling potentially unsafe drinking water.

In discussing the government's role in health care financing, it is useful to consider the categories of health care (De Ferranti 1985): curative care, preventive care that is patient related, and preventive care that is not patient related (see table 2–5). The area in which it seems most reasonable to provide health care services free of charge is in preventive services not related to particular patients. The argument is a very practical one: since no direct transaction takes place between the supplier of the service and any particular clients, as in the case of pest control, it is not feasible to charge individuals who benefit from the service. If a fee were charged there would be no way of limiting the benefits to those who choose to pay. Because of the nonexclusivity of the service, it is argued that a public agent should provide the service, with the cost being covered from general revenues (taxes).

There is, in principle, no difficulty in charging the cost of patient-related preventive care to the patient. The child being immunized or the woman receiving pre- or postnatal care are readily identified. Still, such services are usually provided free of charge or well below actual cost. There are two main arguments for this subsidization. First, certain preventive services, such as measures taken against contagious diseases, create externalities that warrant subsidy. Preventive measures may also reduce disabilities that would represent a burden to the community (for example, prenatal care can prevent low birth weight and the physical or mental disabilities that may accompany it). In such cases, subsidy can be defended on economic grounds.

Table 2-5. Categories of Medical Care

Category	Description
Curative care	Includes personal services (care of patients) rendered by health care facilities and independent providers, including traditional practitioners; and purchases of medicine. Can be subdivided into "first-contact" services (all outpatient) and referral services (inpatient and some outpatient).
Patient-related preventive care	Includes services to well patients—particularly infants, mothers, and pregnant women—delivered through maternal and child health clinics at health care facilities and community health programs. Typical services are immunization, growth monitoring, and instruction on improved breastfeeding and weaning practices.
Nonpatient-related preventive care	Includes disease control (both vector control and mass campaigns), sanitation, education and promotion of health and hygiene, control of pests and zoonotic diseases, and monitoring of disease patterns.

Source: De Ferranti 1985, p. 67.

The second argument for subsidizing patient-related preventive health services is that the population may not be fully aware of the benefits of preventive care, whereas society as a whole (the government) perceives such services to be of great value. Preventive care is thus seen as a merit good, and measures are taken to increase consumption; these measures include launching informational campaigns, granting subsidies, providing the good free of charge, and even rewarding those who decide to consume the good.

The case for subsidizing curative care is by far the weakest. The client is clearly identified and all benefits accrue to him or her. The overriding argument for subsidizing curative care that directly benefits the private consumer is that those in need have a basic right to medical care and that it is socially desirable that they should not face financial or other barriers to such care.

Policies intended to lower these barriers and to provide medical care to those in ill health have taken many forms. The governments of some industrial countries have sponsored programs for certain target groups (in the United States, for example, there is Medicaid for the poor and Medicare for the old). Others have public insurance schemes that cover virtually the entire population (as in the Federal Republic of Germany and the Netherlands) or have nationalized health care systems (as in Canada and the United Kingdom). Similar systems can be found in developing countries, but the dominant way of reducing the financial barrier to obtaining medical care is by direct subsidy, including the provision of health care free of charge.

The Role of Price in the Health Care Market

There is, of course, no such thing as free medical care. The cost has to be borne by somebody. This cost has two aspects: the cost of providing care and the cost of obtaining care. The latter, borne by the consumer, includes not only the fee charged but also the opportunity cost of time used to travel to the health care facility and to wait for service, the actual cost of such travel, and so on. Thus, even when the fee is zero, the private cost is positive (and can be quite large).

The cost of providing medical care is the sum of all inputs, such as wages and salaries of workers and the cost of equipment, drugs, hospital maintenance, and other items. If medical care is financed mostly with general revenues, the health care sector has to compete with other sectors for scarce government resources. Thus, in the aggregate, the health care sector faces a budget constraint, and some form of rationing has to take place even if medical care is provided free of charge.

Many of the problems facing health care systems in the developing world (and in many industrial countries) can be traced to the virtual elimination of price signals in the medical market. On the supply side, investments in both human and nonhuman capital are no longer guided by relative prices and expected benefits. Rather, they are influenced by government subsidies for medical education or stem directly from centrally planned health care programs. Such programs often favor high technology and curative care over low-cost primary care and preventive measures.

On the demand side, consumers no longer face as great a financial barrier to obtaining medical care, but, given that overall resources are limited, other rationing mechanisms have taken the place of the price mechanism. This raises the question of how successful governments have been in increasing access to medical care by subsidizing or providing the goods and services free of charge. Who receives the care? How much? How does the rationing take place in the absence of the price mechanism?

In one study of current methods of financing medical care, the health care sector's inefficiencies are described, as is the effect of these policies on demand (World Bank 1987). The study concludes that governments have not been successful in providing care to those who need it. The better-off in most countries benefit more from free or subsidized services than do the poor. Rural areas in particular are badly served by public health care facilities.

Individuals who need care do not obtain it because, in most developing countries, prices at public medical care facilities are zero or very close to zero. When monetary prices are zero, time prices ration the market and replace monetary prices in determining the choice of medical care provider (Becker 1965; Acton 1975; Dor, Gertler, and van der Gaag 1987; see also Sah 1987). Time prices are the opportunity cost of the time spent obtaining care (such as travel time and waiting time). In many developing countries, medical care facilities are more abundant in urban areas, where the rich are more likely to live. Since there are fewer facilities in rural areas, both travel time and waiting time are usually longer. Moreover, the facilities in urban areas tend to be of higher quality than those in rural areas. Therefore, even if the monetary price is zero, the poor pay higher real prices than the rich do because of the geographic distribution of facilities.

This again leads us to a central question: if the heavy subsidization of medical care in developing countries has not had the desired effect of providing improved access to those in need, what is the alternative?

Furthermore, if governments do not have enough resources to provide adequate medical care to the population, where can additional
resources be found? An answer frequently offered is the reintroduc-
tion of user fees (see, for example, World Bank 1987). Of course the
argument against user fees—that they may present a barrier to medical care—is exactly the reason why subsidies or free medical care
were instituted in the first place. Before such a policy can be implemented a number of questions need to be answered: for which services should fees be charged; how high should charges be; are
patients, especially the poor, willing to pay these charges; and how
much revenue can be raised? The answers depend almost wholly on
the response of consumers to changes in the price of medical care. Is
medical care price elastic? Do patients consider the price of medical
care if they are ill? Will patients still use government health care
services if a fee is charged? Are the poor more price sensitive than the
rich?

Surprisingly, there is little empirical evidence on this subject, especially with reference to the developing world. This book is intended
to fill this gap. In the next chapter we will present descriptive analyses
of the health care infrastructure, health care financing, and health care
utilization patterns in Côte d'Ivoire and Peru. We will demonstrate
that, despite the governments' best intentions (for example, in Peru
the population has the constitutional right to obtain free medical care
from the government), large parts of the population do not have
access to modern medical care. Rationing of limited health services
takes place not through the price mechanism but through geographical distribution and queueing.

Later we will explore the issue of nonprice rationing to formally
define and measure the willingness to pay for medical care. We will
estimate income and price elasticities for medical care and provide
answers to the main questions posed in the foregoing, including those
about the effect of user fees on the poor and the potential for raising
revenues.

Summary

There are several important reasons that governments play a large
role in providing medical care. One is the strong correlation between
economic development and health. Furthermore, if health is seen as
a basic human right, the market alone should not determine the
distribution of medical care. Some characteristics of medical care

(such as uncertainty about when and how much is needed, consumer ignorance, and externalities) justify some form of government intervention or financing. Reducing the cost of medical care to the consumer puts the burden of financing on the government. The severe budgetary constraints faced by many governments in developing countries have caused the results of government policies in the health care sector to fall far short of expectations.

Medical care takes many forms, and the economic arguments for government financing or subsidization are stronger for preventive medical care than they are for curative care. Even for some kinds of preventive care, such as those that directly benefit the client, the benefits of subsidization may not always exceed the economic costs. The case for subsidizing curative care, or providing curative care free of charge, is the weakest, at least on economic grounds. When good health and access to medical care are considered basic rights, however, the social benefits of providing medical care free of charge or at highly subsidized prices may well exceed the economic costs, provided, of course, that such policies succeed in eliminating the barriers to medical care.

In the next chapter we will investigate to what extent the provision of medical care at close to zero cost has succeeded in providing adequate medical care to those who need it, regardless of their ability to pay. We will take a close look at the health care sectors of Côte d'Ivoire, where medical care is provided free of charge, and Peru, where we find a variety of health insurance schemes as well as large government subsidies for most kinds of medical care.

Notes

1. The data of Kravis, Heston, and Summers include information on health care expenditures, adjusted so as to be fully comparable across countries. We will use these data in the next section of this chapter.

2. Cornia, Jolly, and Stewart (1987) provide evidence about the deterioration of nutrition and health status (especially among children) during the first half of the 1980s.

3

The Health Care Systems in Côte d'Ivoire and Peru

In the following chapters we will provide a detailed analysis of the demand for medical care in Côte d'Ivoire and Peru. This chapter presents socioeconomic information that can serve as background for the empirical studies.

Health and Health Care in West Africa

Côte d'Ivoire, situated in West Africa, has about 10 million inhabitants, of which more than 60 percent live in rural areas.

West Africa has some of the poorest countries in the world. Benin, Burkina Faso, and Guinea-Bissau, to name just a few, have per capita incomes well below $400 a year. Health indicators for this region reflect the poverty. Life expectancies at birth are low, especially in Guinea, Guinea-Bissau, and Sierra Leone (table 3–1). Infant mortality rates exceed 150 per thousand for several of the countries in this region and are as high as 175. Child death rates range from 7.3 per thousand in the Congo to 43.5 per thousand in Mali and Sierra Leone.

Other indicators sketch an equally bleak picture. For instance, most of the countries in this region do not produce enough food to match the daily calorie intake requirements of the population. Primary school enrollment in five out of the twenty countries listed is below 50 percent, and the vast majority of the people have no access to clean drinking water.

Table 3–1 also shows basic indicators of the health service infrastructure in these countries. Perhaps the most striking fact is that so little is known. For one third of the countries such simple measures as the population to physician ratio are not available. The data that are available show a large variation, part of which is likely to be the result of differences in definition. In those low-income Sub-Saharan countries for which there are data we find just over one doctor for

Table 3-1. Socioeconomic Indicators for Selected West African Countries

Country or group	GNP per capita (U.S. dollars)	Life expectancy at birth (years)	Infant mortality rate[a]	Child death rate[a]	Percentage of calorie requirements	Primary school enrollment (percent)	Access to safe drinking water (percent)	Population per physician (thousands)	Population per nurse (thousands)	Population per hospital bed (thousands)
Gabon	4,100	50.7	108.3	21.9	122.2	118.0	—	—	—	—
Congo, People's Rep.	1,140	56.9	77.8	7.3	109.2	—	25.0	—	—	—
Cameroon	800	54.5	92.0	10.4	87.5	108.0	—	—	—	—
Nigeria	730	49.6	110.4	21.4	85.7	—	—	12.0	3.0	1.6
Côte d'Ivoire	610	52.4	106.0	15.0	111.5	79.0	65.9	—	—	—
Liberia	470	49.9	128.0	23.2	102.5	76.0	—	9.4	3.2	—
Mauritania	450	46.2	133.0	25.2	97.5	37.0	84.0	—	—	—
Senegal	380	46.2	137.6	27.0	102.4	53.0	42.0	14.2	2.2	—
Ghana	350	52.9	94.8	11.3	65.9	79.0	47.0	39.2	3.3	1.7
Guinea	330	38.4	175.6	30.6	97.0	63.0	10.0	8.1	0.8	0.6
São Tome and Principe	330	64.1	60.9	—	96.8	—	80.0	2.8	0.7	—
Cape Verde	320	64.1	70.2	12.6	88.9	131.0	50.0	6.3	1.0	0.5
Sierra Leone	310	38.4	175.6	43.6	90.5	45.0	16.0	19.3	2.3	0.9
Benin	270	49.0	116.0	18.6	82.9	67.0	20.0	17.0	1.7	1.0
Central African Rep.	260	48.6	138.0	27.2	90.6	77.0	—	23.1	2.1	0.7
Togo	250	52.5	98.4	12.4	93.7	102.0	42.0	21.2	1.9	—
Guinea-Bissau	190	38.4	175.4	30.6	97.0	63.0	10.0	8.1	0.8	0.6
Niger	190	43.3	141.6	28.7	96.6	27.0	33.0	—	—	—
Burkina Faso	160	45.2	145.6	30.4	85.0	27.0	30.0	51.6	3.2	—
Mali	140	45.9	175.6	43.5	68.0	24.0	6.0	27.8	2.5	—

Table 3-1 (continued)

Country or group	GNP per capita (U.S. dollars)	Life expectancy at birth (years)	Infant mortality rate[a]	Child death rate[a]	Percentage of calorie requirements	Primary school enrollment (percent)	Access to safe drinking water (percent)	Population per physician (thousands)	Population per nurse (thousands)	Population per hospital bed (thousands)
Reference groups										
Low-income Sub-Saharan Africa	219.9	48.2	128.5	25.7	90.0	60.1	25.2	39.2	3.3	1.7
Middle-income Sub-Saharan Africa	1,025.3	51.0	103.2	17.6	94.2	98.5	45.8	11.3	2.6	1.4

— = not available.

Note: Countries are listed in order of descending GNP per capita.

a. Per thousand population.

Source: World Bank 1986.

25

every 40,000 people, one nurse for every 3,300 people, and one hospital bed to serve 1,700 people. For middle-income Sub-Saharan countries the situation is somewhat better, especially with regard to physicians.

Though generalizations have a tendency to obscure rather than to illuminate facts, it seems fair to say that the health care system in a typical country in West Africa is poorly developed. Indeed, the averages presented in table 3–1 do not reveal some of the most serious deficiencies of the health care systems, such as the skewed distribution of services in favor of urban areas and the poor quality of the services, such as inadequate equipment and drugs in hospitals and clinics. In general, the lack of a sound financial basis has dried up resources for anything but the salaries of the staff. (See Vogel 1988 for a detailed description of health care financing in four West African countries: Côte d'Ivoire, Ghana, Mali, and Senegal.)

The Ivorian Health Care System

Since it gained independence in 1960, Côte d'Ivoire has seen steady economic growth, from a gross national product (GNP) per capita of $145 in 1960 to $1,207 in 1980, the high point of its economic development. This Ivorian Miracle resulted from an energetic export-oriented economic policy that made Côte d'Ivoire the number one exporter of cocoa in the world and the number two exporter of coffee (den Tuinder 1978). The country's reliance on these two export crops makes it vulnerable to large fluctuations in commodity prices. After the boom in coffee and cocoa prices during the mid-1970s, the coffee price declined 31 percent and the price of cocoa 10 percent during 1977–78. The government tried to keep the economy in high gear by increasing public investment, financed by heavy external borrowing.

The burgeoning external public debt made it clear that this policy could not be continued. A financial recovery and structural adjustment program was initiated in 1981. Public investment was cut by 21 percent, and in 1983 the government's current and capital expenditures were reduced by an additional 20 percent. The initial consequences for the economy were severe. Employment in the modern sector declined 31 percent between 1979 and 1984 (Newman and Lavy 1988). Per capita private consumption declined about 35 percent in real terms during the same period (table 3–2). Although the adjustment measures are beginning to have their intended effect, the outlook over the short run suggests at least a continued stagnation of the economy in terms of gross domestic product (GDP) per capita.

Table 3-2. Macroeconomic Indicators for Côte d'Ivoire, for Selected Years, 1965–84
(billions of CFAF, 1984 constant prices)

Indicator	1965	1970	1975	1980	1981	1982	1983	1984
GDP	1,059.4	1,632.3	2,225.2	3,210.3	3,248.1	3,123.5	2,991.0	2,869.3
GDP per capita (thousands of CFAF)	325.9	415.3	400.9	474.2	379.9	353.6	321.6	293.9
Government expenditure	—	—	332.6	535.2	501.7	496.4	474.8	442.8
Government expenditure as percentage of GDP	—	—	14.9	16.7	15.4	15.8	15.8	15.4

— = not available.
Source: World Bank estimates.

Against this background there is little room for government initia-
tives to improve the health care system of the country. That such an
initiative is called for is evidenced by the current health status of the
population and the status of the country's health care infrastructure.

Since 1960, crude health indicators have improved significantly.
The infant mortality rate decreased from 167 per thousand in 1960 to
119 per thousand in 1980, and life expectancy at birth increased from
39 to 47 years (table 3–3). Still, these indicators are little better than
those prevailing in neighboring West African countries that are much
poorer, and they compare unfavorably to those of an average lower-
middle-income country. Clearly, the development of health care programs has lagged behind that in countries at similar stages of
development.

Large differences in health status exist within the country. In
Abidjan, the capital, estimated life expectancy at birth was 56 years in
1979, compared with only 39 years in the rural savannah regions and
50 years in the urban savannah regions. Child mortality rates in rural
areas were twice as high as in Abidjan. Some of the disparity is likely
to be related to the unequal distribution of welfare in Côte d'Ivoire.
Based on the value of total household consumption, only 3.3 percent
of those in the lowest quintile live in Abidjan, whereas 45.7 percent of
the poorest live in the savannah area (table 3–4). Just 3.9 percent of
the richest quintile live in the savannah, whereas 42.8 percent of them
live in Abidjan. This large urban-rural welfare gap is paralleled by the
distribution of health care facilities.

About 40 percent of the population in Côte d'Ivoire lives in urban
areas. Abidjan alone accounts for a population of 1.6 million, or about

**Table 3-3. Health Indicators for Côte d'Ivoire and
Lower-Middle-Income Countries, 1960 and 1980**

	Côte d'Ivoire		Lower-middle-income countries (average)	
Indicator	1960	1980	1960	1980
Crude death rate[a]	24	17	20	12
Infant mortality rate[a]	167	119	114	89
Child mortality rate[a]	40	23	28	13
Life expectancy at birth (years)	39	47	45	56

a. Per thousand population.
Source: World Bank.

Table 3-4. Regional Distribution of Welfare in Côte d'Ivoire
(*percent*)

Area	Total	Quintile of total household consumption				
		1	2	3	4	5
Abidjan	18.8	3.3	5.2	13.2	29.2	42.8
Other cities	22.4	7.0	18.1	28.2	27.1	31.8
Rural east	24.7	35.2	35.4	22.5	19.9	10.6
Rural west	15.2	8.8	19.6	21.9	14.9	11.0
Rural savannah	18.9	45.7	21.8	14.1	9.0	3.9
Total	100.0	100.0	100.0	100.0	100.0	100.0

Note: Quintile 1 is lowest.
Source: Glewwe 1987a.

17 percent of the total of 9.3 million (these are 1983 figures). All major hospital facilities are in the cities. The two university hospitals (about 1,300 beds altogether) are situated in Abidjan, and the five regional hospitals (general hospitals with about 275 beds apiece) are found in the cities of Bouaké, Man, Daloa, Abengourou, and Korhogo. Together these hospital facilities account for 41 percent of all beds. Rural areas are served by small local hospitals, maternity and child care units, dispensaries, and mobile health units.

Hospitals employ 70 percent of all doctors, 45 percent of all midwives, and more than 50 percent of all nurses. About 60 percent of all doctors are based in Abidjan. Overall, the distribution of medical personnel across occupations is unbalanced. In 1983 there were about 600 doctors, 2,200 nurses, and 1,000 midwives but virtually no skilled auxiliary workers. Given the current system for training health workers, the number of physicians is estimated to increase from 6.5 per 100,000 population in 1983 to 7.8 in 2000. The number of nurses per capita will increase from about 24.9 to 26.5. Thus the already low nurse to doctor ratio of 3.8 will further decrease to about 3.4.

All health workers are paid by the government. Medical care is, in principle, provided free of charge, though some attempts are under way to introduce user fees for hospital care. It is estimated that only 3.1 percent of the total cost of health care is currently covered by user fees (Vogel 1988).

For 1984 the government's budget for health care was CFAF 32.6 billion, or 6.8 percent of the total budget, down from 7.5 percent five years earlier. More than 75 percent of this budget is for personnel cost, about 8 percent for drugs, and the rest for materials, equipment, maintenance, and other operating costs. Projections indicate that the total health budget will soon be insufficient to cover just the cost of personnel, unless the health budget grows much faster than other parts of the government budget or other financial resources are found.

The general quality of the existing health care facilities leaves much to be desired. A 1979 study showed that of the 309 dispensaries one third were more than twenty years old, only 19 percent had piped water, and just 21 percent had a working water pump. Of the 126 mother-child health care units 45 percent had no water and 31 percent no electricity. The two university hospitals in Abidjan have occupancy rates well in excess of 100 percent, but many of the hospitalized patients are just waiting for the arrival of necessary drugs and other supplies or for the repair of equipment.

The most recent data on the population's health status and health care utilization stem from the Côte d'Ivoire Living Standards Survey, conducted in 1985. Based on survey respondents' descriptions of their own health status, about 30 percent of the population suffers from an illness or injury during any given four-week period (table 3–5). No significant sex differentials exist, but there is a distinct age profile. Young children (age zero to five years) show an incidence of illness and injury equal to the overall average, whereas older children (age six to fifteen) show the lowest incidence rate. Adults (sixteen and over) show a monotonic increase of illness with age. There do not appear to be any urban-rural differences in the incidence of illness.

Table 3–6 reflects the anticipated decline in health associated with age: the number of days during which individuals are restricted in their daily activities because of an illness or injury increases with age. The average number of days a month in rural areas during which individuals could not pursue their normal activities is 7.5 for males and 7.9 for females, compared with 5.3 days in urban areas. Although the incidence of self-reported health problems appears to be about the same in rural areas as in the cities (table 3–5), health problems are on average more severe in rural areas.

Table 3–7 shows the distribution of visits to formal health workers, that is, doctors, nurses, and midwives. Since obstetric care is included in the table, it is no surprise that prime-age females usually obtain more medical care than prime-age males. In the two oldest cohorts, in which obstetric care is no longer relevant, the reverse occurs: elderly females obtain less formal care than elderly males, with the exception of women age 36 to 49 living in Abidjan. Although the elderly are less healthy than younger adults, they tend to consume less medical care, particularly in rural areas.

Perhaps the most important result in table 3–7 is that in Abidjan 60 percent of the individuals who report an illness or injury obtain some

Text continues on page 35

Table 3-5. Individuals Reporting an Illness or Injury During the Past Four Weeks in Côte d'Ivoire
(percent)

Age (years)	Abidjan			Other cities			Rural areas			All Côte d'Ivoire		
	Male	Female	Total	Male	Female	Total	Male	Female	Total	Male	Female	Total
0–5	30.7	35.2	33.2	30.3	29.9	30.1	32.0	30.0	31.2	31.5	31.0	31.3
6–15	22.0	20.1	21.0	23.0	20.6	21.8	20.6	19.9	20.3	21.4	21.0	20.3
16–35	26.4	32.9	29.9	27.1	31.6	29.7	24.0	26.8	25.6	25.6	29.4	27.7
36–49	40.8	40.3	40.6	44.8	44.6	44.7	46.1	42.3	43.7	44.6	42.4	43.3
50+	32.1	42.0	35.9	57.5	51.2	54.2	54.8	55.7	55.3	52.8	53.1	53.3
Total	27.8	30.8	29.4	30.4	30.8	30.6	31.0	31.2	31.1	30.3	31.0	30.7

Note: Data are as reported by respondents, for the four weeks preceding the survey.

Table 3-6. Days of Restricted Activity During the Past Four Weeks in Côte d'Ivoire

Age (years)	Abidjan			Other cities			Rural areas			All Côte d'Ivoire		
	Male	Female	Total	Male	Female	Total	Male	Female	Total	Male	Female	Total
0–5	5.6	4.5	4.9	4.7	5.4	5.0	6.1	6.3	6.2	5.7	5.7	5.7
6–15	3.9	4.0	4.0	3.8	3.6	3.7	5.1	4.8	5.0	4.6	4.4	4.5
16–35	3.6	5.5	4.7	3.7	5.6	4.8	7.5	7.3	7.4	5.4	6.4	6.0
36–49	3.9	8.5	6.1	4.5	7.1	5.9	7.5	7.5	6.5	6.1	7.5	6.9
50+	8.4	10.3	9.2	10.2	7.7	9.0	11.0	12.5	11.7	10.7	11.5	11.1
Total	4.5	5.6	5.1	5.0	5.6	5.3	7.5	7.9	7.7	6.4	7.0	6.7

Note: Data are as reported by respondents, for the four weeks preceding the survey.

Table 3-7. Ill or Injured Individuals Who Obtained Medical Care in Côte d'Ivoire
(percent)

Age (years)	Abidjan			Other cities			Rural areas			All Côte d'Ivoire		
	Male	Female	Total	Male	Female	Total	Male	Female	Total	Male	Female	Total
0–5	68.3	69.0	68.7	69.6	60.3	65.0	46.3	41.9	44.4	54.4	51.4	53.0
6–15	50.7	61.6	56.2	50.5	52.1	51.2	41.9	40.9	41.4	45.6	47.6	46.6
16–35	54.0	62.2	58.7	53.9	57.5	55.9	39.6	47.3	44.3	47.5	53.9	51.3
36–49	60.8	68.0	64.4	62.5	59.1	60.7	45.4	38.9	41.5	52.4	47.3	49.5
50+	60.0	47.6	54.4	52.3	46.0	49.2	32.3	31.2	31.8	37.5	34.7	36.1
Total	57.5	63.5	60.8	57.1	55.6	56.3	40.6	40.1	40.3	47.3	48.0	47.6

Figure 3-1. Health Care Utilization by Type of Provider in Côte d'Ivoire
(percent)

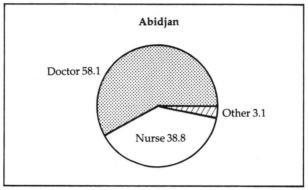

Abidjan

Doctor 58.1

Other 3.1

Nurse 38.8

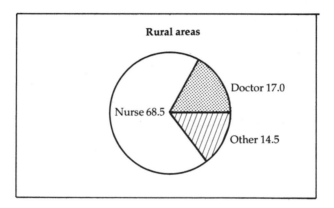

Rural areas

Doctor 17.0

Nurse 68.5

Other 14.5

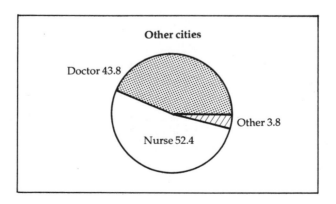

Other cities

Doctor 43.8

Other 3.8

Nurse 52.4

form of medical care, whereas only 40 percent of those living in rural areas do. This quantitative difference in the utilization of health care is aggravated by qualitative differences. Figure 3–1 shows that 58.1 percent of the patients in Abidjan are treated by a physician and 38.8 percent by a nurse. In rural areas only 17.0 percent receive treatment from a physician; the vast majority of the patients, 68.5 percent, see a nurse.

The data illustrate the severity of health problems in Côte d'Ivoire. Roughly one third of the population is ill during any given four-week period, and, on average, those who are ill lose about one quarter of their time because of illness. Utilization of health care is highly skewed in favor of urban dwellers with regard to both quantity and quality. Just 40 percent of the ill in rural areas receive any type of medical care, and most of this is provided by nurses rather than physicians. Cost recovery is virtually nonexistent in Côte d'Ivoire, the health budget is shrinking as a percentage of the total government budget, and the economic outlook for the country shows little if any growth for the foreseeable future. Additional financial resources, other than general government revenues, need to be found, not just to maintain the current situation but to make the significant improvements that are necessary. Introducing user fees is one option. The desirability and feasibility of this option depend on the willingness to pay for medical care. Our analytical work, presented in chapter 5, focuses on the determinants of health care utilization in rural areas, on the basis of which we estimate the willingness to pay for medical care.

Health and Health Care in Latin America

Peru, situated on the west coast of South America, has a population of more than 18 million. With a GNP per capita of about $1,000, the country is considerably better off than most West African countries. In general, GNP per capita in Latin America ranges from $1,000 to $3,410 (Bolivia, with a GNP per capita of $540, is the exception; see table 3–8).

The health indicators are also well above those in West Africa. (See World Health Organization 1982 for a more extensive evaluation of health status in Latin America. See also Zschock 1980 and 1983, Cox and Geletkanycz 1977 for details on Peru.) Life expectancy at birth in an average middle-income Latin American country is 65.6 years, compared with 51.0 years for a middle-income Sub-Saharan African country. The average infant mortality rate is 56.1 per thousand and

Table 3-8. Socioeconomic Indicators for Selected Latin American Countries

Country or group	GNP per capita (U.S. dollars)	Life expectancy at birth (years)	Infant mortality rate[a]	Child death rate[a]	Percentage of calorie requirements	Primary school enrollment (percent)	Access to safe drinking water (percent)	Population per physician (thousands)	Population per nurse (thousands)	Population per hospital bed (thousands)
Venezuela	3,410	69.4	37.8	1.6	99.2	105.0	81.0	1.0	0.5	0.3
Argentina	2,230	70.1	34.4	1.3	119.2	107.0	57.0	0.5	0.6	0.2
Uruguay	1,980	73.3	28.8	0.9	99.1	109.0	80.0	0.5	0.7	0.2
Brazil	1,720	64.1	67.8	5.5	106.0	102.0	71.0	1.3	1.2	0.3
Chile	1,700	70.1	21.8	0.5	105.5	111.0	84.0	1.0	0.5	0.3
Colombia	1,390	64.7	48.4	2.7	109.7	120.0	92.0	2.1	1.0	0.6
Paraguay	1,240	65.8	43.8	2.2	121.7	103.0	21.0	1.4	0.7	0.7
Ecuador	1,150	65.0	67.2	5.4	89.2	115.0	51.8	2.1	1.1	0.6
Peru	1,000	59.3	94.6	11.2	85.0	116.0	51.0	1.7	0.9	0.5
Bolivia	430	52.5	118.4	19.5	81.8	87.0	37.0	2.0	2.7	0.5
Reference group Middle-income Latin America and Caribbean	1,782	65.6	56.1	4.3	109.3	107.3	66.3	1.3	1.2	0.4

Note: Countries are listed in order of descending GNP per capita.
a. Per thousand population.
Source: World Bank 1986.

the child death rate is 4.3 per thousand, compared with 103.2 and 17.6 for middle-income Sub-Saharan African countries. Primary school enrollment is virtually universal, but one third of the population still has no access to safe drinking water.

As for the health care infrastructure, there is on average one physician for every 1,300 people and about an equal proportion of nurses. There is one hospital bed for every 400 people.

Thus both the health indicators and the data on the health care infrastructure are considerably more favorable in Latin America than in Sub-Saharan Africa. This is in keeping with the fact that most Latin American countries are middle-income countries. Still, the state of health and medical care in Latin America has much room for improvement. For instance, although the infant mortality rate has seen a steady decrease, its absolute value of 56.1 per thousand is well above the rates usually found in industrial countries. Moreover, most infant deaths still occur because of communicable diseases. The Pan American Health Organization (1982) reports that 24 percent of all deaths of children between the ages of one and four in Latin America resulted from infectious and parasitic diseases that are preventable by immunization.

Unequal access of urban and rural dwellers to medical care is a significant problem. In Colombia, for instance, an estimated 6 million people, or half the population, do not have access to primary care (Zschock 1979). In the battle over the scarce financial resources available for medical care, urban hospitals have won over rural primary care facilities and preventive activities.

The Peruvian Health Care System

Peru's economic growth during the past twenty years has been shaped by two completely different strategies for managing the economy: a period of nationalistic popular reforms from 1968 to 1975 followed by a period of stabilization, structural adjustment, and liberalization from 1975 to 1985.[1]

During the first period, a self-proclaimed Revolutionary Government of the Armed Forces seized power and promised to implement drastic social reforms such as nationalization, agrarian reform, educational reform, worker participation in the management of firms, and promotion of cooperatives and "social property." It introduced subsidies for oil, gasoline, and staple foods; prices of other basic products were also controlled or heavily subsidized.

The second period began in 1975 with a coup d'état against the reformist military government. A group of more conservative militarists seized power and called for a return to a more orthodox management of the economy, with more reliance on the private sector. In an attempt to reduce government deficits and disequilibrium in the external sector, the new government drastically reduced subsidies and dismantled several social reforms of the preceding period. The government was committed to a program of stabilization and economic growth according to a free market strategy. A new civilian government came to power in 1980. Without changing the basic orientation in the management of the economy, this government began consecutive drastic but unsuccessful stabilization programs. It also began a medium-term strategy of structural adjustment leading toward trade liberalization.

Data in table 3–9 show the behavior of some macroeconomic aggregates during the two periods. During the popular reforms of 1970–75 the average annual rate of GDP growth was 4.8 percent, slightly below the historically high rate of 5.5 percent in the 1950s and 1960s. Population grew at 2.7 percent a year, and per capita income increased at an average rate of 2.0 percent. Also during this period, annual inflation rose from a historically low rate of about 5 percent to 13 percent in 1975 and 30 percent in 1976.

During the adjustment and liberalization of 1975–85 the population growth rate declined to 2.6 percent, but the average annual rate of GDP growth dropped to 1.2 percent; per capita income declined by an average rate of 1.2 percent a year. Inflation skyrocketed from 30 percent during the mid-1970s to 59 percent in 1980, 110 percent in 1984, and 170 percent in 1985. Economic recession was particularly severe during the last five years of the structural adjustment and trade liberalization programs.

Between 1980 and 1985 the economy remained almost stagnant; GDP fell at a rate of 0.7 percent a year, and per capita income declined even faster, at 3.4 percent a year. In 1985 income per capita was about 6 percent lower than at the beginning of the 1970s.

During the first phase of the military government, after two years of austerity measures and policy reform (1969–70), the government pursued expansionary fiscal policies. Government expenditures as a proportion of GDP increased from an average of 16 to 18 percent during previous years to more than 20 percent during the early 1980s (table 3–10). Revenues did not increase in proportion, and domestic and foreign borrowing were heavily used to finance rising government deficits.

These deficits, which were about 3 to 4 percent of GDP between 1971 and 1974, increased to 6 percent in 1976 and 7.5 percent in 1977. The government then attempted to control expenditures. Favorable ex-

Table 3-9. GDP, Inflation, Population, and Income for Peru, for Selected Years, 1970–85

Item	1970	1975	1980	1981	1982	1983	1984	1985
Real GDP (billions of 1980 U.S. dollars)	6.2	12.2	14.5	16.7	14.4	11.1	10.0	14.2
Annual growth rate (real terms, percent)	5.0	–0.5	0.1	3.1	0.6	–12.5	4.4	1.9
Inflation rate (percent)	5.0	13.0	59.2	75.4	64.4	111.2	110.2	169.9
Population (millions)	12.8	14.6	16.6	17.0	17.4	17.9	18.4	18.9
Income index (1970 = 100; real terms)	100.0	110.7	113.9	114.6	112.8	95.9	97.4	96.7

Source: Suarez-Berenguela 1988.

Table 3-10. Public Sector Finances in Peru, for Selected Years, 1970–85

(millions of intis)

Item	1970	1975	1980	1981	1982	1983	1984	1985
Central government								
Expenditure	42.1	106.7	1,046.7	1,830.2	2,634.0	6,048.0	10,728.3	23,869.0
Revenue	38.8	88.6	1,008.4	1,509.7	2,459.6	3,732.0	5,228.1	21,667.0
Deficit	–3.3	–18.1	–38.3	–320.5	–174.4	–2,316.0	–5,500.2	–2,202.0
Total government								
Expenditure as share of GDP (percent)	17.5	19.4	21.1	22.1	19.1	23.9	18.8	15.4
Deficit as share of GDP (percent)	–1.4	–3.3	–0.8	–3.9	–1.3	–9.1	–9.6	–1.4

Source: Suarez-Berenguela 1988.

port prices, resulting in additional export tax earnings, were used in part to balance the budget. Thus the government deficit as a percentage of GDP was reduced to 4.7 percent in 1978, 0.5 percent in 1979, and 0.8 percent in 1980.

During the 1980s, amid structural adjustment and liberalization, inconsistent expansionary fiscal and monetary policies were pursued. From 1980 to 1984 high government expenditures continued; in 1984 total government expenditures represented almost 24 percent of GDP. An unsuccessful reform of the tax system and the economic recession resulting from worsening terms of trade led to a drastic reduction of government revenues. The deficit rose sharply from 0.8 percent of GDP in 1980 to more than 9 percent in 1983 and 1984.

Increases in government expenditures have not been uniform for all government functions. Between 1973 and 1981 the most important changes were reductions in the share of government expenditures on such social programs as health, education, housing, and community activities. Expenditures for these social programs declined from approximately one third of the total budget in 1973–75 to less than one fifth in 1981. In 1981 a single item—"other purposes"—absorbed the largest proportion of government expenditures. This item comprises mainly the interest and amortization payments on domestic and foreign public debt. Debt-related payments increased from 10 percent of government expenditures in 1973 to 21 percent in 1981. Estimates for 1984–85 show that these payments represented 25 to 27 percent of government expenditures.

The overall picture of the 1980s is that of a government struggling to stabilize the economy. The budgetary pressures are such that increasing the outlays for social services is virtually out of the question. The return of the economy to the path of sustained economic growth, so elusive during the 1980s, is still not in sight.

The implications of these developments for the health care sector could be severe. Despite major progress during the past decades, much remains to be done to improve the health status of the population. Table 3–11 shows the movement of health indicators over the period from 1950 to 1986. In 1986 average life expectancy at birth was estimated at 60.8 years, below the average of 61.2 years for other Latin American countries and the average of 71 years for industrial countries.

Like most developing countries, Peru experienced a significant increase in life expectancy during the 1950s and 1960s, and the rate of growth leveled off between 1975 and 1985. Cumulative increases in life expectancy declined from 13 percent between 1960 and 1970 to less than 5 percent between 1975 and 1985. Life expectancy at birth leveled off in industrial countries only after it reached seventy years.

Data also show that whereas both birth and mortality rates have been declining, infant mortality remains high, which is the primary explanation for the relatively low life expectancy and still high crude mortality rates. Peru's infant mortality rate is about 90 per thousand; it is one of the highest among Latin American countries and is in sharp contrast to the infant mortality rates of the most developed countries, whose rates range from 10 to 20 per thousand.

Given the economic outlook, it is unlikely that much improvement in these health indicators can be expected to result from the overall improvement of living conditions that is associated with economic growth. Rather, improved medical care is called for, if not to increase the health status of the population then at least to maintain it at current levels even if there should be a further decline in the economy.

Again, the primary question is where to find the resources to pay for maintaining and, indeed, improving the present health care system. Currently, the Peruvian system is a combination of both governmental and nongovernmental programs and institutions. In 1983–84 the public health sector, comprising all institutions providing both preventive and curative health services to the general public, had 116 hospitals, 463 health centers, and 1,405 health posts (table 3–12). Though access to these services is generally free of charge, availability varies by region and there are other forms of nonprice rationing, such as the degree of availability. This effectively means that only an estimated 57 percent of the population has access to public health care. The corporate sector (mainly social security funds, the army, the police, state-owned firms, and agricultural cooperatives) covers about 17 percent of the population.

Although most policy debates on financing health programs concentrate on financing the public health sector, this sector's expendi-

Table 3-11. Health Indicators for Peru, for Selected Years, 1950–86

Indicator	1950–55	1975	1980–85	1986
Crude birthrate[a]	47.0	39.4	37.0	35.0
Crude mortality rate[a]	21.6	12.2	11.7	9.7
Infant mortality rate[b]	156.0	106.6	99.0	90.5
Fertility rate[c]	—	5.6	4.9	4.7
Life expectancy at birth (years)	44.1	56.5	58.9	60.8

— = not available.
a. Per thousand population.
b. Live birth, up to one year.
c. Births per woman of child-bearing age.
Source: Suarez-Berenguela 1988.

tures represent only about 10 percent of total health care expenditures (table 3–13). Expenditures of the corporate health sector and private households on health-related goods and services represent about 90 percent of total expenditures. These results show a further need to explore the potential role of the corporate and private sectors in implementing health care programs.

Still, more than half of the population has to rely on public health services, not counting the estimated 25 percent of the population that has effectively no access to any form of medical care.

Lack of access is a direct result of the skewed geographical distribution of health care facilities. Hospitals are concentrated in the Lima metropolitan area and other major cities. Health centers and health posts are better distributed, but shortages are still evident, especially in the more remote rural areas (Carrillo 1986). Moreover, health facilities in rural areas show a high degree of deterioration. For instance, in the Cuzco and Cajamarca regions health facilities function at less than 50 percent of capacity because of deteriorated equipment, and 80 percent of the health posts do not have water and sewerage facilities (Carrillo 1986, p. 19).

Table 3-12. Health Care Facilities in Peru, by Sector, 1983–84

Sector	Hospitals	Health centers	Health posts	Other	Percentage of population covered
Public	116	463	1,405	13	56.5
Corporate	98	149	130	0	16.6
Private	116	18	3	4	1.8
Total	330	630	1,538	17	74.9

Source: Suarez-Berenguela 1988.

Table 3-13. Health Care Expenditures in Peru, by Sector, 1980–84

Sector	Expenditure per capita (U.S. dollars)	Expenditure as percentage of GDP	Expenditure as percentage of total
Public	10–17	0.6–0.8	10
Corporate	100–130	2.3–3.1	45
Private	11–20	2.1–3.5	45
Total	55–77	5.0–7.0	100

Source: Suarez-Berenguela 1988.

The skewed distribution of health care facilities mimics the overall distribution of welfare. Average per capita income in Lima was 771 intis a month in 1985–86, but in the rural sierra it was less than half that (table 3–14). Only 6 percent of the poorest quintile live in the Lima metropolitan area, and more than 50 percent live in the rural sierra, though the population of both areas is approximately the same.

Tables 3–15 and 3–16 show the percentage of people who report an illness or injury and the number of restricted days of those who are ill. The patterns are similar to those in Côte d'Ivoire: the incidence is higher in urban areas, but illness is more severe in rural areas.

Almost half of the ill or injured in Lima receive some form of medical care, whereas less than 30 percent receive care in rural areas (table 3–17). The difference in quantity is aggravated by differences in quality. More than 85 percent of medical care in Lima is provided by doctors, whereas less than half of the rural population receives medical care from physicians (see figure 3–2).

In sum, the evidence supports a call for significant improvements in the Peruvian health care system, especially in rural areas. At the same time, the economic outlook raises the questions of whether there will be government resources to make those improvements and whether health care would be the best use of scarce resources. The large differences between health care in urban and rural areas suggest that redistributing resources would partly improve the rural health care system. The introduction of user fees may be another option.

Summary

There are a number of similarities between the health care systems of Côte d'Ivoire and Peru. First, in both countries the government provides medical care free of charge. In Peru, the corporate and private sectors complement the public sector in urban areas, but in rural areas the population still has to rely on government-provided services. Second, the economic situation in both countries severely constrains the government budget, making it all but impossible to provide the resources to expand the medical system. Third, most public services accrue to the better-off urban dwellers, whereas the rural population has limited access to public facilities. Moreover, the quality of these facilities leaves much to be desired.

Obviously, additional resources are necessary to provide medical care of sufficient quality to rural areas, but these resources are not available in the government's budget. Are user fees the answer? For urban areas, or, more precisely, for better-off households in urban

Text continues on page 50

Table 3-14. Regional Distribution of Welfare in Peru
(*percent*)

Area	Total	Quintile of total household consumption					Mean expenditure per capita (intis a month)
		1	*2*	*3*	*4*	*5*	
Lima	26.8	6.0	18.2	28.8	35.4	45.5	770.9
Urban coastal	15.2	11.1	14.7	17.6	15.4	17.2	569.8
Rural coastal	7.2	8.8	9.8	7.2	6.8	3.5	421.3
Urban sierra	11.0	9.0	9.6	10.2	11.5	14.8	649.9
Rural sierra	30.5	52.8	38.5	28.1	22.9	10.4	366.8
Urban forest	3.0	2.1	2.8	2.3	3.0	4.7	792.0
Rural forest	6.3	10.3	6.5	5.8	3.9	3.9	413.5
Total	100.0	100.0	100.0	100.0	100.0	100.0	n.a.

n.a. = not applicable.
Note: Quintile 1 is lowest.
Source: Glewwe 1987b.

Table 3-15. Individuals Reporting an Illness or Injury During the Past Four Weeks in Peru

(percent)

Age (years)	Lima			Other cities			Rural areas			All		
	Male	Female	Total	Male	Female	Total	Male	Female	Total	Male	Female	Total
0–5	62.2	64.1	63.2	49.5	50.6	50.1	41.7	42.6	42.1	47.6	49.2	48.4
6–15	40.4	45.2	42.7	30.9	33.1	32.0	29.6	32.4	31.0	32.4	35.5	33.9
16–35	40.1	47.6	44.0	32.8	39.5	36.3	32.1	36.5	34.4	34.9	40.9	38.0
36–49	47.2	60.3	54.2	40.7	52.0	46.5	41.4	53.5	47.5	42.7	55.1	49.1
50+	51.7	62.8	57.5	46.4	64.0	55.5	57.6	65.5	61.9	53.3	64.4	59.0
Total	45.4	53.0	49.3	37.5	44.2	40.5	38.0	43.0	40.5	39.8	46.0	42.9

Note: Data are as reported by respondents, for the four weeks preceding the survey.

Table 3-16. Days of Restricted Activity During the Past Four Weeks in Peru

Age (years)	Lima			Other cities			Rural areas			All		
	Male	Female	Total	Male	Female	Total	Male	Female	Total	Male	Female	Total
0–5	2.1	1.8	2.0	2.5	2.3	2.4	3.1	3.0	3.0	2.7	2.5	2.6
6–15	1.6	1.1	1.4	1.3	1.4	1.4	2.0	2.0	2.0	1.7	1.6	1.6
16–35	1.4	1.3	1.3	1.9	1.6	1.7	2.3	2.1	2.2	1.9	1.7	1.7
36–49	1.7	1.9	1.8	1.8	1.7	1.8	2.9	2.6	2.7	2.3	2.1	2.2
50+	1.6	3.1	2.4	2.4	3.5	3.1	4.0	3.5	3.7	3.1	3.4	3.2
Total	1.6	1.7	1.7	2.0	2.1	2.0	2.8	2.6	2.7	2.3	2.2	2.3

Note: Data are as reported by respondents, for the four weeks preceding the survey.

Table 3-17. Ill or Injured Individuals Who Obtained Medical Care in Peru
(percent)

Age (years)	Lima			Other cities			Rural areas			All		
	Male	Female	Total	Male	Female	Total	Male	Female	Total	Male	Female	Total
0–5	58.8	56.8	57.8	53.4	53.7	53.5	31.3	29.7	30.6	44.0	43.5	43.7
6–15	49.3	36.5	42.7	32.9	38.5	35.7	26.1	21.7	23.8	34.5	30.3	32.4
16–35	47.0	44.0	45.3	45.5	45.9	45.7	30.9	29.3	30.0	40.8	39.5	40.1
36–49	43.0	54.4	49.8	52.5	50.6	51.4	33.0	34.4	33.8	40.9	44.8	43.1
50+	53.5	55.5	54.6	51.2	47.0	48.7	32.9	30.2	31.4	42.1	40.8	41.3
Total	49.9	48.1	48.9	46.0	46.6	46.3	30.6	28.8	29.6	40.3	39.4	39.8

Figure 3-2. Health Care Utilization by Type of Provider in Peru
(percent)

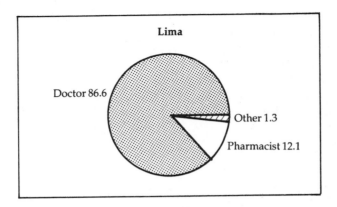

Lima

Doctor 86.6

Other 1.3

Pharmacist 12.1

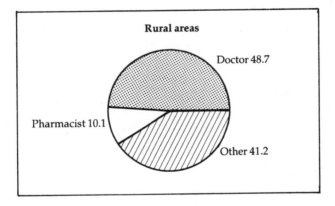

Rural areas

Doctor 48.7

Pharmacist 10.1

Other 41.2

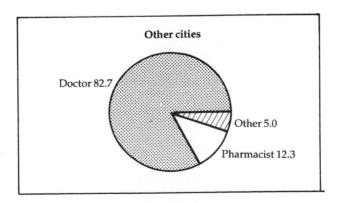

Other cities

Doctor 82.7

Other 5.0

Pharmacist 12.3

areas, the answer to this question seems clear. Given that there are very limited resources for providing medical care, and that there are no clear arguments in favor of across-the-board subsidies for curative care, it makes sense to charge those consumers who can afford it for medical goods and services provided by the government, especially for curative care. Public resources thus saved could be used to help upgrade rural health care facilities and subsidize care for the rural poor. But should user fees also be charged at rural primary care facilities? In the rest of this book we will try to answer this question.

Note

1. This section draws heavily on Suarez-Berenguela 1988. We are very grateful to him for permission to incorporate his material.

4

Analytical Issues
in Health Care Financing

Health care systems in the developing world face a multitude of problems that cannot be solved overnight. Governments must consider how much to spend on medical care as opposed to, say, education or railroads; the appropriate mix of public and private funding of medical care; the apparent need to shift resources from curative to preventive care; the most appropriate curricula for health workers; the implications of drug imports for the balance of payments situation; and many other issues. High on the list of problems that need urgent attention is the question of how to finance medical care. How can sufficient resources be generated to maintain a health care system of acceptable quality without putting up financial barriers that deny access to the system to all but the richest few? This is the issue addressed in the rest of this book, with emphasis on curative primary care in rural areas.

This chapter discusses how various aspects of this problem can be approached analytically. We consider options for resource mobilization and especially the pros and cons of introducing prices (user fees). We will show, in general terms, how concerns for equity and efficiency can be addressed empirically if we improve our knowledge of the determinants of the demand for medical care, especially regarding the effects of income and prices.

We present the framework used by economists in analyzing welfare; provide a formal definition of the willingness to pay for medical care; and show how, armed with a properly specified model of the demand for medical care, we can answer such questions as how much revenue can be raised and who wins or loses under various policies.

Options for Health Care Financing

The health care systems of Côte d'Ivoire and Peru are in poor shape partly because of the way they are financed. In this respect these two countries are not exceptional. Problems in the health care systems of developing countries can be said to arise from flaws in three areas: allocation (not enough funds are spent on cost-effective health programs); internal efficiency (public programs are wasteful or of poor quality); and equity (health services are inequitably distributed) (World Bank 1987, p. 13).

This study goes on to identify the fundamental cause of these problems as "poor approaches to financing." As we have seen, the vast majority of financial resources for health services comes from government revenues or other general funds (such as social security plans; see also Jimenez 1987, Katz 1987). Only a tiny fraction of the cost is recovered from direct payments by consumers. If one could count on sustained economic growth, a rapid increase in the government budget for health care might help to sustain the current health care infrastructure, to make the necessary improvements in quality, and to expand the system to meet the needs of the growing and aging population. The economic outlook of most developing countries, however, shows sluggish growth at best, whereas the global reevaluation of the role of governments in the process of economic development calls for less rather than more government expenditure.

Thus the question is not whether resources other than government revenues need to be found to strengthen the financial basis of the health care system, but where and how. When government funds are insufficient to provide medical care for those in need, there is only one alternative: charge the consumer.

This dichotomy between medical care financed by the government and that financed by user fees is somewhat artificial. First, the government needs revenues to cover its expenditures, revenues it obtains by taxing citizens. Second, consumers can pay for the goods and services in various ways, either directly, at the time of consumption, or through prepaid private insurance or compulsory public insurance schemes. If, in the latter case, health care is provided free of charge, the difference to the consumer between government-financed and privately paid (but fully insured) medical care is negligible. Indeed, such a system is likely to suffer from many of the same problems that characterize a government-financed system. Still, prices can play a role in the fully insured health system, for instance as incentives to the provider to improve efficiency.

In sum, there is a continuum: on one end is a system that is completely financed by the government, in which prices do not play a role; on the other end is a completely market-oriented system, in which prices are used by consumers and producers to allocate the scarce resources available for medical care. We will use the fully government-funded health care system as an extreme case and compare it with one in which additional revenues are raised through user charges.

This study is not concerned with the effect of prices on the suppliers of medical care but rather with the effect of prices on the consumer. Money prices faced by the consumer can be changed by increasing or decreasing government subsidies or by altering the insurance coverage. But, as we will argue, money prices are not the only relevant cost to the consumer; other costs—such as travel cost and time spent traveling and waiting—also are important.

Are user fees a desirable alternative to government revenues for financing medical care? The answer to this question depends on attitudes toward how user fees affect equity and efficiency. These attitudes in turn reflect the government's preferences and how it provides for social welfare. It is unlikely that such attitudes can be determined empirically with reasonable precision. What can be determined empirically is the likely effect on equity and efficiency of a policy that introduces user fees or reduces subsidies in a system that previously provided medical care free of charge or at highly subsidized prices.

The first set of questions that needs to be answered is: How do patterns of demand change as a result of such a policy? Will people make more or less use of certain health care providers? Who will opt out of the system, either by not consuming medical care at all or by substituting, that is, by turning to private providers?

The second set of questions pertains to the consequences of the policies for welfare (again, from the consumer's point of view). In which cases will welfare be increased or decreased by the fee policies? Are the poor more or less affected than the rich? Are there options to offset the negative effects on welfare?

Third, we need to address the question of resource mobilization. Since user fees are proposed because of the paucity of financial resources for health care, the question arises whether those fees can be set high enough to raise enough revenue to improve the health care system.

The answers to all these questions depend on consumers' reactions to such policies. To be more precise, if prices are irrelevant for the consumption of medical care, that is, if patients demand medical care when they need it, regardless of the economic costs, it makes eminent sense to set the fees equal to their marginal costs. In that case one can recover all costs without negative implications for welfare.[1] This, of course, is an unrealistic example. Consumers are sensitive to prices, even in the case of medical care (that is exactly why medical care is provided free of charge or at subsidized prices).

Thus the questions boil down to how sensitive consumers are to price changes, how this differs among households with different incomes, and which other determinants of the demand for medical care are important and can, perhaps, be used to offset some of the negative effects.

The Welfare Analysis of Health Care Demand

In an analysis of economic welfare, the starting point is a decisionmaking unit that, given limited resources and other constraints, tries to maximize its own welfare. This unit is usually an individual or a household, but the general theory can be applied equally well to a government, a firm, or a hospital. If the unit is a firm, welfare could be equated with profits, which are observable. In that case, the problem is one of maximizing profit. If the unit is a household or individual, welfare is less easily defined. Indeed, analysts make do with a vague notion of welfare, or utility, that is not measurable but is assumed to be derived from the consumption of goods and services. In its most general form goods and services can include leisure or savings but also such intangibles as good health. Consequently, the empirical counterpart of this theoretical framework is the consumption of a bundle of goods and services that contributes to welfare either directly or indirectly because, for instance, the goods and services contribute to good health, which in turn contributes to welfare.

Households are assumed to choose the bundle of goods and services that maximizes their welfare. The constraint they face is their command over limited resources. Furthermore, they are guided in their choices by the relative prices of the available goods and services. The analyst observes the household's consumption, the household's total income, and the prices in the market. Given the theoretical framework used in analyzing the maximization of welfare, these data suffice to infer the relative well-being of the households and thus how these welfare levels change under various policy scenarios. These scenarios usually take the form of a change in relative prices or a change in income. We will show that prices should be interpreted broadly to include, for instance, the cost of time spent to obtain the good. But first we will formalize this general framework for welfare analyses.

We will denote a vector of K goods and services as $x = (x_1, x_2, \ldots, x_K)$. Their respective prices are $p = (p_1, p_2, \ldots, p_K)$, and a household's total income is Y. Households are assumed to maximize a utility function U, defined over a bundle of goods and services x, when prices are p and income is Y. In formula:

(1)

$$\max_{x} U = U(x_1, x_2, \ldots, x_K)$$

$$\text{subject to } Y = \sum_{i=1}^{K} p_i x_i \,.$$

The budget constraint says that total expenditures cannot exceed total income.

The result of this maximization problem is the bundle of goods and services chosen by the household. The amount of each item consumed depends in general on income and all prices. This set of demand equations can be written as follows:

(2)

$$x_1^0 = x_1(Y, p_1, p_2, \ldots, p_K)$$

$$x_i^0 = x_i(Y, p_1, p_2, \ldots, p_K)$$

$$x_K^0 = x_K(Y, p_1, p_2, \ldots, p_K) \,,$$

where x_i^0 denotes the optimal quantity of consumption item i.

Substituting (2) into the utility function (1) yields a so-called indirect utility function:

(3)

$$U^0 = U^0(Y, p_1, p_2, \ldots, p_K).$$

This function shows the maximum welfare level, U^0, that can be reached with income Y, when prices are p. The most useful tool for welfare analyses is the inverse of this function:

(4)

$$Y = C(U^0, p_1, p_2, \ldots, p_K).$$

This function, called a cost function, shows how much income, Y, is needed to obtain a given welfare level, U^0, when prices are p.

Since this cost function answers the question of how much it costs (how much income is needed) to obtain a given welfare level when prices are, say, p^0, it can also show how much more it will cost if prices rise to p^1. Thus, with the use of equation (4), we can calculate the additional income a household needs to stay at the same welfare level when prices move from p^0 to p^1. This amount is known in the economic literature as the compensating variation (see, for example, Deaton and Muellbauer 1980).

Let us compare two situations. The only difference between the two is a change in the price of good i from p_i^0 to p_i^1. Before the price change the cost function reads

(5)
$$Y^0 = C\,(U^0, p_1, p_2, \ldots, p_i^0, \ldots, p_K).$$

After the price change we have

(6)
$$Y^1 = C\,(U^0, p_1, p_2, \ldots, p_i^1, \ldots, p_K).$$

To compensate a household for the welfare loss incurred by raising one of the prices, we need to pay the household the amount $(Y^1 - Y^0)$, the compensating variation. We will now show how this theoretical framework can be used to address the main questions of this study.

Let p_f be the fee for obtaining medical care and p_t be the sum of all other costs (travel time, waiting time, travel costs, and so on). Then

(7)
$$p_m = p_f + p_t\,,$$

where p_m is the total cost of medical care.

Equation (7), simple as it is, will play an important role in our analyses. First of all, as we will show in chapter 5, it will allow us to obtain price elasticities for medical care even when p_f, the user fee, is zero. Second, it will allow us to address such questions as: If we increase the fee for care, p_f, how can we compensate for the corresponding welfare loss (for example, by reducing various aspects of p_t)? The issue of compensating for welfare loss will be addressed with the help of equation (4), the cost function.

If p_i^0 in equation (5) represents the total cost for medical care, that is, the sum of the fee p_f and the private costs p_t, and p_i^1 in equation (6) is the new total cost, resulting from the reduction in p_t and increase in p_f, then $(Y^1 - Y^0)$ is the amount of money that leaves the household equally well off in both situations. In other words, the compensating variation $(Y^1 - Y^0)$ is the maximum amount a household is willing to pay for the improved access (reduced travel time, for example) to a clinic or hospital.

This notion of willingness to pay must be introduced to discuss the effects on welfare and the potential for generating revenue of introducing or increasing user fees for social services. The willingness to pay should be distinguished from the ability to pay. The idea of ability to pay is sometimes used regarding the consumption of other goods, mostly luxuries such as alcohol and theater tickets. As long as a person's expenditures on such luxuries exceed the expected costs of medical care, it is judged that he or she is able to pay for medical care.

Unfortunately, someone's ability to pay is only relevant for evaluations of policy if one can coerce the person into consuming the goods or services. In the more common situation, in which one has to rely on people's choices, we can infer from observed consumption patterns only whether one is willing to pay for the goods or services.

This is where the empirical work begins: with the observation of consumption patterns, that is, with the estimation of the system of demand equations given in (2). Of course, many factors other than income and price influence the demand for goods and services. For instance, if households are analyzed, the size of each household needs to be taken into account. If a specific item, such as medical care, is analyzed, such factors as education, sex, and the age of the individual will play a role. If we denote all such intervening variables by $h = (h_1, h_2, \ldots, h_L)$, we can write the vector of demand equations as

$$(8) \qquad\qquad x = x\,(Y,p;h).$$

This system of demand equations can be estimated from household survey data, provided that sufficient variation in the price vector p is observed. That is often not the case. As already noted, however, prices should be interpreted broadly; the cost of obtaining medical care includes not only the fee paid to the doctor but also the time and cost of traveling to the clinic or hospital. These costs are specific to the household or the individual. Thus, even when money prices (fees) are the same for all individuals, the total cost of obtaining care is likely to vary. This variation in individuals' cost of obtaining medical care allows us to estimate price responses even if money prices are zero. Subsequently, the price responses will allow us to perform the necessary analysis of welfare, as already outlined.

As we discussed in chapter 2, the consumption of medical care can yield substantial positive results, especially the prevention of communicable diseases. This suggests that an analysis of individuals' willingness to pay for medical care does not capture the total improvement in social welfare gained by improving the medical care system. Since our study focuses on the willingness to pay for curative treatment, we believe that private compensating variations capture most of the welfare measurement.

Summary

Certain economic tools are needed to answer questions about the effect of user fees on the demand for medical care, on welfare, and on the budget. One such tool, part of the theoretical framework used in analyzing the effects of policies, is a precise definition of the willingness to pay for medical care. Willingness to pay, and not ability to pay, is the appropriate criterion for judging the feasibility and desirability of alternative pricing policies.

The theoretical framework also serves as a guide for empirical work. First, observations on current patterns of consumption of medical care can be used to estimate demand equations to quantify the influence of such variables as income, price (including, for example, travel time), education, and family size, among other things. These demand equations can then be used to calculate price elasticities that show how price-sensitive consumers are and how price sensitivity differs among consumer groups. Given this empirical evidence, the tools of welfare economics can be used to quantify the implications for welfare and the budget of various policy scenarios.

Note

1. Marginal cost pricing will not lead to full cost recovery under increasing returns to scale. In this case, Ramsey pricing would be appropriate (see, for example, Baumol and Bradford 1970).

5
Modeling the Demand for Health Care

Evaluation of the feasibility and desirability of user fees requires a preevaluation of the consequences for health care utilization, revenue, and welfare. This, in turn, requires knowledge of the properties of the demand function, especially price elasticities and the effect of other nonmonetary costs such as travel time. The price elasticities provide information about how user fees will affect utilization and revenues. Knowledge of the effects of travel time can be used to measure the amount individuals are willing to pay for improved access (reduced travel time). If governments open new health care facilities in rural areas (thus making people better off by improving access), then the willingness to pay is linked to the maximum price that can be charged for these facilities without making individuals worse off.

The usually straightforward exercise of estimating demand is greatly complicated in the case of health care by the fact that there is often little or no variation in price within a country. In many developing countries most medical services are run by governments, which set prices close to or, in many cases, equal to zero. Even when prices are positive, they are typically uniform within the country. A second complication in modeling the demand for medical care is that the decision to use services is discrete. Individuals choose whether to visit a clinic, hospital, or private doctor or not to obtain care at all (that is, they treat themselves). A third issue, and one that is not restricted to medical care, is that the effects of user fees are likely to vary by income so that the distributional consequences must be considered. Indeed, if the poor are more price-sensitive than richer individuals, user fees will reduce the utilization by the poor more than by the rich. In such a case, uniform user fees would be regressive.

In this chapter we derive a discrete choice specification of the demand for medical care from a utility-maximizing theoretical model. We also show how private time-price variation can be used to identify the parameters necessary to compute price elasticities and measures of willingness to pay (these are called compensating variations). The model makes use of the well-known result that private prices, such as the opportunity cost of time, ration the market when monetary prices are absent or small (Becker 1965). An added advantage of the model is that the theoretical framework naturally leads to an empirical specification that is flexible enough to allow the price elasticities and measures of willingness to pay to vary by income level.

In our model we focus on the decision to seek care and the choice of provider. In studies on the utilization of medical care in industrial countries, most notably the Rand Corporation's health insurance experiment (Manning and others 1987), researchers focus on the determinants of how much medical care individuals choose to consume, given that they seek care, as well as the decision to seek care at all. Indeed, Manning and others find that price affects the decision to seek care. We focus on the effect of prices on the decision to seek care because the policy question we seek to address is: To what extent do prices (user fees) prevent individuals from seeking care? We believe that this is appropriate given that the policy debate in the industrial world concerns how to reduce the overconsumption of medical care, whereas the dilemma in the developing world is how to find a financing mechanism that does not reduce access—indeed, that increases access—to good medical care.

In this chapter we review the literature on the demand for medical care, derive a theoretical model of choice of medical care provider, and specify that model's empirical counterpart.

Evidence from the Literature

The literature on the demand for medical care in developing countries contains conflicting messages. One camp suggests that prices are not important determinants of utilization of medical care. Akin and others (1984, 1986); Schwartz, Akin, and Popkin (1988); Birdsall and Chuhan (1986); and Heller (1982) report very small and sometimes positive price effects, most of which are statistically insignificant. Another body of work—by, among others, Mwabu (1986, 1988); Gertler, Locay, and Sanderson (1987); Alderman and Gertler (1988); and Cretin and others (1988)—concludes that prices are important. All of these studies, except for Cretin and others, employ discrete choice provider models. The study by Cretin and others examined household medical expenditures in China and reported that differences in coinsurance rates explain one third of the variation in expenditures on medical care.

The results of the first group of studies contrast sharply with most recent studies on the demand for medical care in industrial countries, which uniformly conclude that prices are important determinants of utilization of medical care. The most important and comprehensive of these studies is the Rand Corporation's National Health Insurance Study (HIS), which was a five-year controlled, randomized trial experiment conducted in five sites in the United States, involving over 20,000 individuals (Manning and others 1987). The HIS provides overwhelming evidence that prices are statistically significant determinants of utilization of health care. Price elasticities are found to be on the order of –0.2. Moreover, the HIS results are on the low end of the estimates of price elasticity from the nonexperimental literature, which finds statistically significant price elasticities ranging from –0.2 to as high as –2.1 (for examples see Rosset and Huang 1973, Davis and Russel 1972, Phelps and Newhouse 1974, Goldman and Grossman 1978, Colle and Grossman 1978, and Newhouse and Phelps 1974 and 1976).

This divergence between the literature on industrial countries and that on developing countries is somewhat paradoxical. Indeed, prices might be expected to be less important in industrial countries than in developing countries. Two reasons are immediately apparent: (1) income levels are substantially higher in industrial countries, and (2) medical insurance is almost universal in industrial countries and virtually nonexistent in developing countries. Higher income levels and pervasive insurance coverage imply that medical care takes up a much smaller percentage of household budgets in the industrial world than in the developing world. Individuals might be expected to be more sensitive to prices when these prices constitute a bigger share of their budget.

In addition, estimated income elasticities suggest that price elasticities should be higher in developing countries. We know, from the Slutsky decomposition of the price elasticity of demand, that the price elasticity increases with the income elasticity, other things being equal (see, for example, Deaton and Muellbauer 1980). The empirical evidence shows that the demand for medical care is more income elastic in the poorer, developing countries than in the richer, industrial countries. Engel curve estimates for medical care in Birdsall and Chuhan (1986) and Musgrove (1983) report income elasticities close to unity, whereas income elasticities between 0.2 and 0.3 are typically found for industrial countries (see, for example, Van de Ven and van der Gaag 1982, Holtmand and Olsen 1978, Colle and Grossman 1978,

Goldman and Grossman 1978, Phelps 1975, and Manning and others 1987).

In most developing countries, the price of medical care at government-run facilities is small or, in many cases, zero. Hence it is not surprising that prices do not ration the market. Acton (1975) and others have shown that when monetary prices are small, the price of time (that is, the opportunity cost of time used in obtaining the good) rations the market. Time prices could be expected, therefore, to ration the market in developing countries. Indeed, in almost all of the studies on the demand for medical care in developing countries just cited, travel time is an important and significant determinant of demand for medical care. These results suggest that when monetary prices become larger they will begin to ration demand as well.

How then can we explain the paradoxical results of zero price elasticities in developing countries? One explanation is that the models of demand for medical care in developing countries are misspecified. The studies typically model demand as a discrete choice, with the price effect specified to be independent of income. This assumption is restrictive, since one would expect the wealthy to be less sensitive to price differences among providers than the poor. In fact it can be shown that these models are inconsistent with utility maximization (Gertler, Locay, and Sanderson 1987; this point is demonstrated explicitly in the next section). Another possible cause for the paradoxical result is more straightforward. Many of the studies of demand for medical care in developing countries use data sets of dubious quality. The information, especially that on income, prices, and travel time, leaves much to be desired. A final point is that the studies just mentioned specify time prices as nonmonetary nuisance parameters in the utility function, implying that their coefficients reflect the marginal disutility of traveling. Becker (1965) points out that time prices should enter via the budget constraint. Dor, Gertler, and van der Gaag (1987) extend the model of Gertler, Locay, and Sanderson by including time prices in the budget constraint to estimate travel time elasticities. Gertler and van der Gaag (1988) show that variation in travel time is sufficient to identify all of the parameters necessary to compute monetary price elasticities and compensating variations.

The Behavioral Model

Our framework is a model in which utility depends on health and on the consumption of goods other than medical care. If an illness is experienced, individuals decide whether to seek medical care. The benefit from consuming medical care is an expected improvement in health, and the cost of medical care is reduced consumption of other goods and services.

Individuals have to decide not only whether to seek care but also what type of care. They are able to choose from a finite set of alternative providers, one of which is self-treatment. Each provider offers an expected improvement in health (efficacy) for a price. Let us define the quality of an alternative provider as the expected improvement in health as a result of that provider's medical care. The price of an alternative includes both monetary outlays and private access costs such as the opportunity cost of travel time. Taking into account this information and their incomes, individuals choose the alternative that yields the highest expected utility.

Formally, let the expected utility conditional on receiving care from provider j be given by

$$(1) \qquad U_j = U(H_j, C_j) ,$$

where H_j is the expected health status after receiving treatment from provider j and C_j is consumption net of the cost of obtaining care from provider j.

The medical care purchased from provider j is invested in health. The quality of provider j's medical care is defined as the expected improvement in health over the health status that an individual would enjoy if he or she treated him or herself. In essence, quality is defined as an expected marginal product. Let H_0 be the expected health status without professional medical care (with self-treatment). Then the quality of provider j's care is $Q_j = H_j - H_0$, which yields an expected health care production function of the form

$$(2) \qquad H_j = Q_j + H_0.$$

As specified in (2), quality varies by provider and may in fact also vary by individual characteristics such as severity of illness and the educational attainment, age, and sex of the individual.

The health production function assumes a simple form for the self-care alternative. Since $H_j = H_0$, we have $Q_0 = 0$. This implicitly normalizes the health care production function so that the quality of a particular provider's care is measured relative to the efficacy of self-care.

Consumption expenditures (net of expenditures on medical care) are derived from the budget constraint. The total price of medical care includes both the direct payment to the provider and the indirect cost of access (for example, the opportunity cost of travel time). Let P_j^* be the total price of provider j's care and Y be income, so that the budget constraint is

$$(3) \qquad\qquad C_j + P_j^* = Y,$$

with $C_j > 0$ required for the jth alternative to be feasible. Substitution of (3) into (1) for C_j yields the conditional indirect utility function

$$U_j = U(H_j, Y - P_j^*).$$

Notice that income affects utility through the consumption term and that the price of medical care is forgone consumption.

The time spent obtaining care could, in principle, come at the expense of work in the marketplace, production work at home, or leisure. In that case income Y and net consumption C_j should incorporate the value of the three activities. In an economy that is only partially monetized, such as the one in rural Côte d'Ivoire, nontraded home production is a principal source of income. We capture this by including the value of home production consumed by the household in the measure of income. Adding the value of leisure, however, would greatly complicate the model and is left for future work. Hence we implicitly assume that lost time comes at the expense of work or home production and not at the expense of leisure. The measurement of income is discussed in chapter 6.

We are now ready to specify the utility maximization problem. Suppose the individual has $J + 1$ feasible alternatives (with the $J = 0$ alternative being self-care). The unconditional utility maximization problem is

$$(4) \qquad\qquad U^* = \max (U_0, U_1, \dots, U_J),$$

where U^* is maximum utility. The solution to (4) gives the alternative that is chosen and, when there are random terms in the model, the probability that each alternative is chosen. The probability an alternative is chosen can be interpreted as the demand function in a discrete choice model. These demand functions, then, can be used to solve for the unconditional indirect utility functions and the expenditures or cost functions. The unconditional functions can be used to assess the effect of policy changes on welfare.

In summary, individuals who experience an accident or illness are faced with a choice of obtaining treatment from one of several available providers or caring for themselves. Each alternative provider offers an expected improvement in health (quality) for a price that reduces income available for the consumption of nonmedical goods. The individual chooses the provider whose combination of quality and price offers the highest utility, where utility is derived from health and the consumption of all goods and services other than medical care.

Empirical Specifications

The solution to equation (4) yields a system of demand functions whose forms are probabilities that the alternatives are chosen. The probability that a particular alternative is chosen equals the probability that this choice yields the highest utility among all the alternatives. The functional form of the demand functions depends on the functional form of the conditional utility function and the distribution of the stochastic variables.

The Conditional Utility Function

Gertler, Locay, and Sanderson (1987) show that income can influence the choice of provider only if the conditional utility function allows for a nonconstant marginal rate of substitution of health for consumption. This point is easily demonstrated by an example in which two alternatives are available. Suppose that the individual has the choice between self-care and doctor-provided care and that the conditional utility function is linear, which imposes a constant marginal rate of substitution. Thus the utility from doctor-provided care (denoted by subscript d) is

$$U_d = \alpha_0 H_d + \alpha_1 (Y - P_d)$$

and the utility from self-care (subscript s) is

$$U_s = \alpha_0 H_s + \alpha_1 Y.$$

Then the individual chooses doctor-provided care if

(5) $$U_d - U_s = \alpha_0 (H_d - H_0) - \alpha_1 P_d > 0.$$

If the alternative of doctor-provided care is chosen, the individual experiences an improvement in health of $(H_d - H_s)$ and a reduction in nonmedical consumption of P_d. If the individual chooses doctor-provided care, he or she gets an increase in utility of $\alpha_0 (H_d - H_0)$ from improved health and a reduction in utility of $\alpha_1 P_d$ from reduced consumption. The decision rule in (5) says that the individual will choose doctor care if the net change in utility is positive.

Equation (5) also shows that if the marginal utility of health and the marginal utility of consumption are constant for all levels of income (that is, if there is a constant marginal rate of substitution between health and income), then income does not contribute to which alternative is chosen. This is indicated by the fact that Y differences out of (5).

Some studies on the choice of health care provider try to include income in the model by specifying linear utility functions with alternative specific coefficients on income (Akin and others 1984 and 1986; Schwartz, Akin, and Popkin 1988; Birdsall and Chuhan 1986; Dor and van der Gaag 1987; and Mwabu 1986). This specification is inconsistent with stable utility maximization. For instance, consider our earlier example, with the exception that the coefficients on consumption vary by alternative:

$$U_d = \alpha_0 H_d + \alpha_{1d}(Y - P_d)$$

and

$$U_s = \alpha_0 H_0 + \alpha_{1s}Y.$$

Notice that the marginal utility of consumption is constant but varies by alternative. In this case, doctor-provided care is chosen if

$$U_d - U_s = \alpha_0(H_d - H_s) - \alpha_{1d}P_d + (\alpha_{1d} - \alpha_{1s})Y > 0.$$

In this specification income does not difference out of the decision rule and therefore influences the choice. The identifying restriction, though, is that the coefficient on consumption must be different in the two alternatives. In other words, the marginal utility of consumption must be different for the two alternatives even when evaluated at the same level of consumption. This implies that two alternatives that provide the same improvement in health for the same price must yield different levels of utility to the same individual. If this is true, then preferences are not ordered and transitive, and stable utility functions, therefore, do not exist.

Alternatively, if the functional form does not impose a constant marginal rate of substitution on the conditional utility function, income will influence the choice. To make this point we generalize our example so that the decision rule in (5) is

$$U_d - U_s = U(H_d, Y - P_d) - U(H_0, Y).$$

The income effect is found by the partial derivative

(6) $$\frac{\partial(U_d - U_s)}{\partial Y} = \frac{\partial U(H_d, Y - P_d)}{\partial C} - \frac{\partial U(H_0, Y)}{\partial C}.$$

If the derivative of the conditional utility function with respect to consumption, $\partial U/\partial C$, is constant (that is, $\partial^2 U/\partial C^2$ and $\partial^2 U/\partial C\partial H$ are zero), then (6) is zero and income does not influence the choice. When

$\partial U/\partial C$ is nonconstant, (6) is nonzero and income does influence the choice. Also, the marginal rate of substitution, $-(\partial U/\partial H)/(\partial U/\partial C)$, is nonconstant when $\partial U/\partial C$ is nonconstant.

Another implication of the model is that if health is a normal good, the effect of price is smaller for larger incomes. This point requires the reasonable assumption that $\partial U^2/\partial C\partial H \geq 0$ (that is, that the marginal utility of consumption increases with improved health). For health to be a normal good, (6) must be positive. For (6) to be positive $\partial^2 U/\partial C^2$ must be negative; that is, the conditional utility function must be concave in consumption. Now we use this information to show that the effect of price diminishes with increases in income. The price effect is

$$\frac{\partial(U_d - U_s)}{\partial P} = -\frac{\partial U(H_d, Y - P_d)}{\partial C}.$$

Thus an increase in income influences the price effect by

$$\frac{\partial^2(U_d - U_s)}{\partial P\partial Y} = -\frac{\partial U^2(H_d, Y - P_d)}{\partial C^2}.$$

Hence an increase in income reduces the negative effect of price if $\partial^2 U/\partial C^2$ is negative. Therefore, if health is a normal good (that is, $\partial^2 U/\partial C^2 < 0$), the effect of price on the choice diminishes with income.

This point can be made in a more intuitive context. If health is a normal good, then the demand for health increases with income. A necessary condition for normality is that as income rises the marginal rate of substitution of consumption for health diminishes, holding health constant. This point is demonstrated in figure 5–1, where the case of continuous choice, with health being a normal good, is depicted. As income rises, the point of utility maximization moves out from the origin along the expansion path. With health constant at $\overline{H}$, the point moves to the right along the horizontal line as income rises, intersecting the indifference curves at points of flatter slopes, implying a diminishing marginal rate of substitution.

In a discrete choice situation, normality implies that as income rises individuals are more likely to choose the options offering higher price and higher quality. Here, too, a necessary condition for normality is that as income rises the marginal rate of substitution of consumption for health diminishes, holding health constant. This is demonstrated in figure 5–2, where the discrete choice case, with health as a normal good, is depicted. In figure 5–2, there is a choice between a high price–high quality option (P_H, Q_H) and a low price–low quality option (P_L, Q_L). At a low income level, say Y_L, the choice is between points A

and B, that is, between a gain in health of $(H_H - H_L)$ and a gain in consumption of $(P_H - P_L)$. At income Y_L, the additional consumption is preferred to the additional health, and the low price–low quality option, B, is chosen. The high-income individual with income Y_H has a choice between options C and D. These points represent the same tradeoff between health and consumption as options A and B. As income rises the marginal rate of substitution of consumption for health falls along both horizontal lines H_H and H_L. Eventually, at some income between Y_L and Y_H, the gain in health is preferred to the gain in consumption. At income Y_H, the high price–high quality option, C, is chosen.

In summary, if health is a normal good, then higher-income individuals will choose the high price–high quality option, and lower-income individuals will choose the low price–low quality option, other things being equal. In other words, the price difference dissuades low-income individuals from choosing the high price–high quality option, but it does not dissuade high-income individuals. What matters in the choice is the share of medical care in the household's budget. For low-income individuals the high price–high quality option represents a significant portion of their budget. Rather than give up, say, food, they choose the low price–low quality option. Alterna-

Figure 5-1. The Tradeoff between Health and Consumption: The Continuous Choice Case

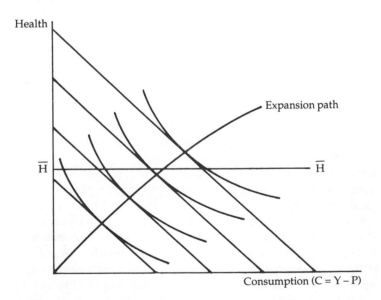

Health

Expansion path

$\overline{H}$ $\overline{H}$

Consumption (C = Y – P)

Figure 5-2. The Tradeoff between Health and Consumption: The Discrete Choice Case

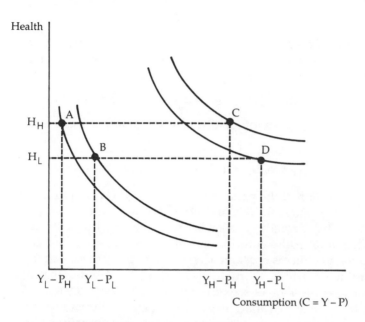

Consumption (C = Y − P)

tively, the high price–high quality option is a small portion of high-income individuals' budgets, implying that they do not have to give up much to choose it. Finally, to allow health to be a normal good and therefore allow income to influence the choice, the functional form of the conditional utility function should not impose a constant marginal rate of substitution. Whether health is a normal good is an empirical question, and the functional form should be flexible enough for the data to answer this question.

A parsimonious functional form for the conditional utility function that does not impose a constant marginal rate of substitution and is consistent with stable utility maximization is the semiquadratic, which is linear in health and quadratic in consumption. Specifically, let the conditional utility function be

$$(8) \qquad U_j = \alpha_0 H_j + \alpha_1 C_j + \alpha_2 C_j^2 + \varepsilon_j,$$

where ε_j is a zero mean random taste disturbance with finite variance and is uncorrelated across individuals and alternatives.

Consumption (that is, income net of the cost of obtaining care from provider j) is derived from the budget constraint in (3). Specifically, $C_j = Y - P_j^*$. The full price of medical care is the direct payment to the provider plus the value of time spent in obtaining the care. Consumption, then, is

(9) $$C_j = Y - (P_j + wT_j),$$

where P_j is the direct payment to provider j, w is the opportunity cost of time, and T_j is the time spent obtaining care from provider j. Substitution of (9) into (8) yields

(10) $$U_j = \alpha_0 H_j + \alpha_1[Y - (P_j + wT_j)] + \alpha_2[Y - (P_j + wT_j)]^2 + \varepsilon_j.$$

Since $P_0 = H_0 = 0$, the conditional utility function for the self-care alternative is

(11) $$U_0 = \alpha_0 H_0 + \alpha_1 Y + \alpha_2 Y^2 + \varepsilon_0.$$

The identification of the parameters in (10) and (11) requires that the values of expected health and consumption differ across the alternatives. The alternative chosen is the one that yields the highest utility. Therefore, if the contribution of either expected health or consumption to utility is constant across alternatives, these variables cannot influence which alternative is chosen. Attributes that are constant across alternatives are differenced out of the decision rule. This implies that it is variation in prices across alternatives that identifies α_1 and α_2. If prices did not vary across alternatives, consumption would be constant across alternatives and difference out of the decision rule.

At this point it is easy to show that all of the parameters can still be identified if monetary prices are zero. The identification of α_1 and α_2 in (10) and (11) requires variation in prices or travel time, or both, across alternatives so that the contribution of consumption varies across alternatives. Hence variation in T_j across alternatives suffices to identify these parameters.

Finally, a simple transformation of the conditional utility function illuminates the role of prices and income in the model. Since the decision rule involves comparing utility levels across alternatives, the conditional utility functions can be normalized relative to one of the alternatives without loss of generality. To illustrate the role of prices and income, we normalize the utility from the self-treatment alternative to zero by subtracting (11) from (10). In this case (5) becomes:

$$U_j - U_0 = \alpha_0 Q_j - \alpha_1 P_j + \alpha_2(P_j^2 - 2YP_j) + \varepsilon_j - \varepsilon_0.$$

Notice that income has differenced out of the consumption term but not out of the consumption squared term. The linear consumption term represents only price, whereas the consumption squared term includes both a price-income interaction term and a squared price term. Thus our specification includes a price term and a price-income interaction. Therefore, if α_2 is not significantly different from zero, income does not influence the choice (that is, the utility function exhibits a constant marginal rate of substitution of health for consumption). Prices do not influence the choice if both α_1 and α_2 are not significantly different from zero.

Quality

The remaining issue in the specification of the conditional utility function is the measurement of the expected efficacy (quality) of each alternative. Substitution of the health production function (2) into the conditional utility function (10) yields

$$(12) \qquad U_j = \alpha_0 H_0 + \alpha_0 Q_j + \alpha_1(Y - P_j - wT_j)$$

$$+ \alpha_2(Y - P_j + wT_j)^2 + \varepsilon_j.$$

Since $Q_0 = 0$, the conditional utility function in (13) for the self-care alternative reduces to

$$(13) \qquad U_0 = \alpha_0 H_0 + \alpha_1 Y + \alpha_2 Y^2 + \varepsilon_0.$$

The $\alpha_0 H_0$ term appears in all of the conditional utility functions, and its value is constant across alternatives. Since only differences in utility matter, these terms can be ignored.

Estimation is complicated by the problem that quality is unobserved in the nonself-care conditional utility functions in (12). We solve this problem by letting Q_j be a parametric function of its observable determinants. The expected quality of provider j's care is the expected improvement in health (marginal product) over the expected level of health that would occur from self-treatment. The expected improvement in health can be viewed as being produced through a household production function. The arguments of the household production function are provider characteristics and individual characteristics such as severity of illness and ability to implement the recommended treatment plan. For example, the expected improvement in health from hospital care relative to self-care may be increasing with educational level, since individuals with higher education may be better able to implement recommended treatment plans.

Moreover, the marginal utility of an individual's health may also vary with household characteristics. For example, the marginal utility of the health of a child may depend on how many children there are in the household. In general, the value of health may vary with many demographic variables such as age, sex, education, and family composition.

The basic determinants of both the quality household production function and the marginal utility of quality are demographic variables. Pollak and Wachter (1975) argue that the distinct effects of demographic variables in the household production function and in the marginal utility of quality cannot be identified separately. Therefore, we specify a reduced form model that shows how utility is derived from quality. Formally, let this function be given by

(14) $$\alpha_0 Q_j = \beta_{0j} + \beta_{1j} X + \eta_j,$$

where X is a vector of the determinants of quality and utility from quality, and η_j is a zero mean random disturbance with finite variance.

To make the specification as general as possible, we let the coefficients in (14) vary by alternative. Allowing for different intercepts permits the baseline quality to vary by alternative, and having different slope coefficients allows the provider's productivity relative to self-care to vary with individual characteristics such as age, education, and severity of illness. The random disturbance term captures unmeasured portions of the quality function. These disturbances may be correlated across alternatives.

Since $Q_0 = 0$, the utility from quality function simplifies to $\alpha_0 Q_0 = 0$ for the self-care alternative. Hence the coefficients in (14) are interpreted relative to the self-care alternative. Notice further that the normalization sets the unobserved portion of quality in the self-care alternative, η_0, equal to zero as well.

Substituting (14) into the conditional utility functions in (12) and ignoring the $\alpha_0 H_0$ term, which appears in all of the conditional utility functions, gives

(15) $$U_j = V_j + \eta_j + \varepsilon_j,$$

where

(16) $\quad V_j = \beta_{0j} + \beta_{1j} X + \alpha_1(Y - P_j - wT_j) + \alpha_2(Y - P_j + wT_j)^2.$

This completes the specification of the indirect conditional utility functions. Notice that the intercept and coefficients on the demographic variables vary by alternative, whereas the coefficients on the economic variables are constant across alternatives. Further, the disturbances in the nonself-care conditional utility functions are correlated with each other, but, since $Q_0 = 0$, they are uncorrelated with the disturbance in the self-care conditional utility function.

The Demand Functions and Welfare

The demand function for a provider is the probability that the utility from that alternative is higher than the utility from any of the other alternatives. Most of the previous studies on the demand for medical care in developing countries have assumed that these demand functions take on a multinomial logit (MNL) form. As discussed in McFadden (1981), the MNL suffers from the assumption of the independence of irrelevant alternatives. This assumption is equivalent to assuming that stochastic portions of the conditional utility functions are uncorrelated across alternatives, and it imposes the restriction that the cross-price elasticities are the same across all alternatives. A computationally feasible generalization of the MNL is the nested multinomial logit (NMNL), which was introduced by McFadden (1981). The NMNL allows for correlation across subgroups of alternatives and, therefore, nonconstant cross-price elasticities. The NMNL allows the grouping of more similar alternatives (closer substitutes) so that the cross-price elasticities are more elastic within groups than across groups. The NMNL also provides a specification test for groupings. The NMNL relates the assumption of the independence of irrelevant alternatives across groups but not within groups. Furthermore, the NMNL is a generalization of the MNL, since the MNL is nested within it. This provides us with a specification test for the MNL.

A more general specification, which does not impose any restrictions on the cross-price elasticities, would require the estimation of multinomial probit (MNP) models. These models are computationally very difficult when there are more than three choices. The NMNL is a computationally tractable compromise between the very restrictive MNL and the MNP. Moreover, the NMNL provides a specification test to determine whether the data reject the functional form and distributional assumptions.

The NMNL specification for our problem is as follows. Following McFadden, we assume that the joint distribution of the η_i's and ε_i is a type B extreme value distribution. Let choice 0 be the self-care alternative, and choice $1, \ldots, J$ be the various provider alternatives. The η_j's imply that the error terms of the provider alternatives may be correlated with each other but not with the self-care alternative. Therefore, the self-care demand function (that is, the probability of choosing self-care) is

$$\pi_0 = \frac{\exp(V_0)}{\exp(V_0) + \left[\sum_{j=i}^{J} \exp(V_j/\sigma) \right]^\sigma},$$

and the demand for provider i is

$$\pi_i = (1 - \pi_0) \left[\frac{\exp(V_i/\sigma)}{\sum\limits_{j=1}^{J} \exp(V_j/\sigma)} \right],$$

where σ is a measure of the similarity of grouped alternatives introduced by the η_j's.

The log likelihood function for this problem is simply

$$\ln L_i = \sum_{j=0}^{J} D_{ij} \ln \pi_{ij},$$

where D_{ij} is a dichotomous variable that takes on the value 1 if individual i chose alternative j. Although a two-step estimate exists (McFadden 1981), we will employ full information maximum likelihood to estimate the model. Hensher (1986) shows that full information maximum likelihood estimation of NMNL yields substantial efficiency gains over the more popular two-step procedure.

McFadden (1981) shows that σ must be between zero and 1 for the model to be consistent with utility maximization. When σ is close to zero, the error terms in the provider alternatives' conditional utility functions are highly correlated. This implies that individuals view providers as closer substitutes for one another than they do any of the providers as substitutes for self-care. Regarding cross-price elasticities, this implies that a provider's demand is more sensitive to another provider's change in price than is self-care demand. Thus if σ is less than 1, an increase in one provider's price will cause a greater percentage increase in other providers' demands than in self-care.

Finally, as already mentioned, the MNL is a special case of the NMNL. Specifically, when σ equals 1, the NMNL reduces to an MNL. In this case the error terms are uncorrelated and the self-care alternative and the providers are viewed as equally close substitutes for one another. Moreover, the cross-price elasticities are constant across alternatives. This condition provides a formal specification test of the MNL.

In general, the value of σ provides us with a specification test. If its values are greater than 1 or less than zero, the data reject either the distributional assumptions or the functional form of the utility function.

The estimated demand functions can be used to project the effect of user fees on demand and revenues and on the number of people who do not seek health care because user fees exist. These demand functions also form the basis of our measurement of the willingness to pay for reduced travel time to a medical care facility. The measure of willingness to pay is calculated as a compensating variation, which is the amount of income that an individual must earn to make him or her just as well off after a price change as before the change. The effect of a price change on welfare involves both an income effect (reduction in $Y - P$) and a substitution effect (changes in the probabilities that the alternatives are chosen). Both must be taken into account in calculating the compensating variation. The calculation involves solving the demand functions to obtain the unconditional indirect utility and expenditure functions with which experiments on compensating variation can be conducted. Small and Rosen (1981) provide the general theory for discrete choice demand systems. Consider changing the vector of travel times to providers from T to T'. In the case of an NMNL, the amount of income that an individual must be given or is willing to forgo to make him as well off at T' as he or she was at T—that is, the compensating variation, CV—is

$$(17) \qquad CV = (1/\lambda) \{ \ln [\exp (V_0) + \left[\sum_{j=1}^{J} \exp (V_j/\sigma) \right]^{\sigma}]$$

$$- \ln [\exp (V'_0) + \left[\sum_{j=1}^{J} \exp (V'_j/\sigma) \right]^{\sigma}]\}$$

where V_j and V'_j are evaluated at T and T', respectively, and where λ is the marginal utility of income.

In order for (17) to be exact, the marginal utility of income λ must be independent of alternative specific characteristics and price (McFadden 1981, Small and Rosen 1981). Although λ is independent of quality, it is not independent of price. Specifically,

$$\lambda = \partial U/\partial Y = \alpha_1 + 2\alpha_2(Y - P).$$

As long as the prices are very small relative to income, λ is likely to be approximately constant across small differences in price. Hence each individual's average marginal utility of income over the alternatives is a good approximation of λ. Although this is little variation in λ for an individual across alternatives, λ may vary greatly across individuals since there is substantial variation in income.

Summary

There is an apparent paradox in the literature on health economics: price elasticities in developing countries are reported to be lower than in industrial countries. There are various reasons for expecting the opposite to hold true. Moreover, theoretical and empirical shortcomings exist in the literature on the demand for health care in developing countries.

We derive a fairly general model of the demand for medical care, based on these points, that has the following attractive properties:

- It is consistent with utility maximization, which allows us to use the derived demand functions for welfare analysis.
- It is flexible. In particular, the effect of price on the demand for medical care is allowed to differ by income level.
- It is empirically tractable.

These properties allow us to answer the main empirical question of this study: How price elastic is the demand for medical care?

6
Estimation and Results

The main purpose of estimating the model of medical care provider choice is to obtain price elasticities of demand so as to be able to investigate the implications for cost recovery, utilization, and welfare of various user fee policies. The estimation results for Peru and Côte d'Ivoire and for all age groups show that prices are important determinants of utilization of medical care. Moreover, as expected, we find that the price elasticity of demand falls with income. Demand is in the elastic range for the lowest income groups, whereas it is inelastic in the upper income groups. These results imply that user fees can generate substantial revenue without much effect on utilization by individuals in the upper income groups, but they may cause large reductions in utilization by individuals in the lower income groups.

The implications of these results for policy and overall welfare will be explored in detail in the next chapter. In this chapter we describe the data and the estimation results for Côte d'Ivoire and Peru. We begin by discussing the provider choices available given the institutional structure of each country, along with the measurement of the variables that are used in the estimation. Then we present the estimated coefficients and price elasticities.

The models are estimated with data from the 1985 Côte d'Ivoire Living Standards Survey and the 1985–86 Peruvian Living Standards Survey. These identical multipurpose household surveys were designed to measure socioeconomic factors relevant to the standard of living. Researchers collected detailed information on individuals' illnesses and utilization of medical care over the four weeks immediately preceding the interview, in addition to many socioeconomic variables relevant to the demand for medical care, such as income, family structure, and education. A useful feature of the Living Standards Surveys is that they also collected community-level information in rural areas. For each village, researchers collected information on travel time to the nearest available medical facility of every type and on village-level agricultural wage rates for males and females.

To ensure flexibility in the empirical specification, separate models are estimated for children and adults in both countries. All of the models are estimated by full information maximum likelihood.

In the appendix to this chapter, we use our data to estimate the misspecified model used in earlier work (Akin and others 1984 and 1986, Birdsall and Chuhan 1986, Dor and van der Gaag 1988, Mwabu 1986, and Schwartz, Akin, and Popkin 1988). The results indicate that prices are statistically significant determinants of the choice of medical provider. This suggests that poor data may have been the reason some studies have not found significant price effects. Since, as pointed out in chapter 5, these models are inconsistent with utility maximization, the results cannot be interpreted structurally. Therefore, the estimates are not representative of demand function parameters.

Rural Côte d'Ivoire

In rural Côte d'Ivoire almost no private health care is available, and few people report using it. The vast majority of individuals who experience an illness or accident seek care initially from a government hospital or clinic, or they do not obtain any professional medical treatment at all. Traditional healers do exist, but less than 3 percent of the people report obtaining traditional care; we leave them out of the analysis. Finally, only a handful of people in rural areas travel the very long distance to an urban area to go to a private doctor or to a pharmacy. Given this information, the relevant medical care alternatives for residents of rural Côte d'Ivoire appear to be government hospitals, government clinics, and self-care. The distribution of choices of health care provider in our sample is given in figure 6–1. This represents the initial choice of provider. Of the 42 percent of individuals who seek professional medical care for an illness, about two thirds go to clinics and one third to hospital outpatient centers.

It is this split of the sample (those who do not seek care, those who go to a hospital, and those who visit a clinic) that we try to explain with our theoretical model. For ease of reference, we repeat this model here. Let π_j be the probability that an individual chooses alternative j, with $j = 0$ being the self-care alternative. Then

$$\pi_0 = \cfrac{\exp(V_0)}{\exp(V_0) + \left[\displaystyle\sum_{j=1}^{J} \exp(V_j/\sigma)\right]^{\sigma}}$$

and

$$\pi_i = (1 - \pi_0) \cfrac{\exp(V_i/\sigma)}{\left[\displaystyle\sum_{j=1}^{J} \exp(V_j/\sigma)\right]^{\sigma}}$$

and σ is 1 minus the correlation between the error terms of the provider alternatives (self-care excluded). Thus the model is specified as a nested multinomial logit (NMNL) model that collapses into a multinomial logit (MNL) model if we find that $\sigma = 1.00$. The term V_j represents the utility derived from alternative j and is parameterized as

$$V_j = \beta_{0j} + \beta_{1j}X + \alpha_1(Y - P_j - wT_j) + \alpha_2(Y - P_j - wT_j)^2,$$

where X is a vector of socioeconomic variables, Y is total income, P_j is the fee for provider j, w is the opportunity cost of time, and T_j is the travel time to provider j.

Figure 6-1. Health Care Provider Choice in Rural Côte d'Ivoire
(percent)

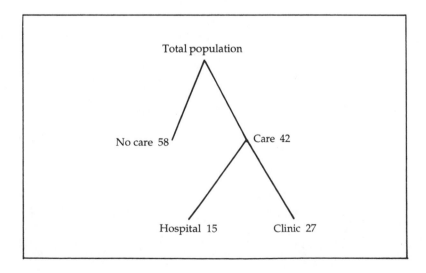

The term $(Y - P_j - wT_j)$, which enters both in linear and quadratic form, shows the effects of income and prices (both monetary and nonmonetary) on the demand for medical care. The vector X includes variables such as age, sex, and education that may influence the efficacy of obtaining care from a specific provider as well as the value (utility) the individual (or household) puts on an increase in health status.

As specified in the theoretical model, an alternative that yields the highest utility is chosen, where utility depends on the expected quality (improvement in health) and on consumption net of medical care. The expected quality and consumption net of medical care must be specified for each option.

Consumption net of medical care is income less the cost of obtaining medical care. Income is calculated as the average monthly value of total household consumption. Household consumption is a better measure of permanent income than reported income because it is less sensitive to temporary fluctuations (such as the seasonality of work) and because it includes the value of home production. In developing countries such as Côte d'Ivoire and Peru, nonmarket activities such as home production are major sources of income (in Côte d'Ivoire the value of home-grown produce consumed by the household amounts to approximately half the food budget and one third of total consumption). Purchasing medical care reduces not only the monetary resources available for other consumption but also the time available for home production and other work.

Since the government facilities had no user fees in 1985, the price of care was the opportunity cost of time spent in obtaining care. Recall from chapter 4 that variation in travel time is sufficient to identify all the parameters of the demand functions, thus allowing calculation of price elasticities and measures of willingness to pay. The opportunity cost of time is calculated as the product of the round-trip travel time and the individual's wage rate.[1] For children, the opportunity cost of the mother's time is used. The round-trip travel time for each individual to each alternative provider comes from the community survey, and the appropriate village-level agricultural wage rate for males and females is taken as the unit opportunity cost of time.

The village-level agricultural wage rates for males and females are reasonable estimates of the opportunity cost of time. Newman (1988) shows that 93 percent of all working adults in rural areas of Côte d'Ivoire are engaged in agricultural activities. Moreover, variation in individual wage rates within a village is likely to be small, since more than 90 percent of the adults have less than one year of schooling.

The utility derived from an expected increase in health status is specified to be a function of the option chosen and individual characteristics. The arguments of the alternative specific functions are individual and family characteristics that may affect quality and the marginal utility of quality. Variables that may influence the efficacy of medical care include age, the number of healthy days last month, education, the number of other adults in the household, and the number of children in the household. Age and the number of healthy days proxy for health status. Age is entered in spline form, with the break occurring at forty years for adults and three for children. The breakpoints were determined by grid searches, which involve finding the breakpoints that maximize the likelihood function. Education (years of schooling) is included because more educated individuals may be better able to implement recommended treatments and therefore produce more health relative to self-care than can less educated individuals. In the case of children the mother's education is used. The family composition variables are included because the more adults and fewer children there are in the household the better able a household may be to self-treat an illness. Variables that may affect the marginal utility of quality include age, sex, and household composition.

Since the vast majority of individuals living in rural Côte d'Ivoire are farmers (97 percent), the sample used for estimation excluded nonfarm households. The sample also excluded households in villages for which community-level information was not available. To focus on primary medical care, visits for obstetric and other preventive purposes were excluded. There were nineteen such cases. The exclusion of villages without community-level data reduced the sample by 8 percent. The final sample included 49 villages, with observations of 1,030 adults and 769 children under the age of 16 who experienced an accident or illness in the four weeks preceding the survey.

Descriptive statistics are presented in table 6–1. We see that 24 percent of the adults and 30 percent of the children who report an illness or injury visit a clinic, and 15 percent of adults and 14 percent of children obtain outpatient hospital care. It is noteworthy that the average travel time is about an hour to clinics and about an hour and three quarters to a hospital.

Estimation Results

The NMNL models of provider choice in rural Côte d'Ivoire were estimated by full information maximum likelihood. One model was

estimated for adults and another for children. The results, presented
in table 6–2, are generally consistent with economic theory.

The estimated value of σ is 0.34 for adults and 0.41 for children. The
estimates are both significantly different from zero and significantly
different from 1. Therefore, the models both are consistent with utility
maximization and reject the MNL specification in favor of the NMNL.
The result that σ is less than 1 also implies that hospital and clinic care
are closer substitutes for one another than are hospital and self-care
or clinic and self-care.

In both the adults' and children's models the coefficients on the
consumption and its square are significantly different from zero. The
signs of the coefficients indicate that the conditional utility function
is concave in consumption. In other words, the marginal utility of
consumption is diminishing but does not become negative in the
relevant range. Prices enter the model via the consumption terms. As
shown in chapter 5, if the prices did not vary across alternatives, the
coefficients on consumption would not be identified, since the value

Table 6-1. Descriptive Statistics for Rural Côte d'Ivoire

	Adults		Children	
Variable	Mean	Standard deviation	Mean	Standard deviation
Clinic[a]	0.24	0.49	0.30	0.55
Hospital[a]	0.15	0.38	0.14	0.37
Clinic travel time[b]	1.18	1.32	0.92	1.16
Hospital travel time[b]	1.90	0.92	1.56	1.60
Monthly family income[c]	97.85	81.19	108.41	99.66
Hourly wage[d]	75.48	28.54	74.89	26.42
Age (years)	44.85	17.12	6.33	3.64
Male[a]	0.46	0.50	0.51	0.50
Education (years of schooling)	0.85	2.16	0.91	2.88
Healthy days in past four weeks	18.60	9.94	22.34	7.24
Number of adults in household	4.57	2.96	4.62	3.01
Number of children in household	4.86	2.44	4.97	2.77
Sample size	1,030		769	

a. Binary variable; equals one if alternative is chosen, zero otherwise.
b. Round-trip travel time, in hours.
c. Calculated as total household consumption and reported in thousands of 1985
Ivorian CFAFs. In 1985, the exchange rate was approximately 461 CFAF to the dollar.
d. 1985 Ivorian CFAFs.

of consumption would then be constant across alternatives. The fact that these coefficients are significant implies that the relative prices of the alternatives are relevant to the choice of the provider. Prices and income enter the model in a highly nonlinear fashion through the consumption terms, making it hard to judge the order of magnitude of their effects. Therefore, we will examine them in detail in the next section. This section is devoted to discussing the effects of the other variables. We begin with the adults and then consider children.

Adults in rural Côte d'Ivoire, unlike those in industrial countries, seem to reduce utilization of medical care over the life span, other things being equal. The coefficients on the first age spline indicate that

Table 6-2. NMNL **Model of Provider Choice Estimates for Rural Côte d'Ivoire**

Variable	Adults		Children	
	Coefficient	t-statistic	Coefficient	t-statistic
Consumption[a]	10.04	5.44	14.43	5.65
Consumption squared[b]	−0.02	3.30	−0.01	2.14
Sigma	0.34	3.54	0.41	4.37
Hospital				
Constant	1.64	1.20	2.68	2.54
Age 1[c]	−0.00	0.11	−0.69	2.31
Age 2[d]	−0.10	2.82	−0.04	0.64
Education	−0.05	0.45	−0.05	0.13
Male	0.73	1.68	0.05	0.13
Children	0.17	2.17	0.21	2.44
Adults	−0.15	1.69	−0.19	2.06
Healthy days	−0.13	3.32	−0.09	2.71
Clinic				
Constant	0.69	0.51	2.50	2.51
Age 1[c]	0.02	0.66	−0.64	2.40
Age 2[d]	−0.10	2.60	0.04	0.76
Education	−0.03	0.31	0.00	0.50
Male	−0.07	0.16	0.17	0.46
Children	0.15	1.89	0.18	2.28
Adults	−0.16	1.78	−0.21	2.30
Healthy days	−0.10	2.45	−0.06	2.05
Sample size	1,030		769	
Log likelihood	−886		−679	

NMNL = nested multinomial logit.
a. Variable divided by 100 for estimation.
b. Variable divided by 100,000 for estimation.
c. Adults age 16–40, children age zero to 3.
d. Adults over age 40, children over age 3.

all individuals between the ages of sixteen and forty are equally likely to seek medical care for the treatment of an accident or illness. After age forty the demand for both hospital care and clinic care falls progressively.

One explanation for this unusual pattern of utilization of medical care over the life span may be derived from human capital theory. Families may prefer to invest scarce resources in the health of members for whom the return is higher. For the same improvement in health, the economic return, measured by family income, is higher from investing in the younger, more productive members of a family than from investing in the elderly. A second reason may be that the available medical care in rural Côte d'Ivoire is best suited to addressing the acute health problems common to adults in their prime rather than the more complex, chronic problems of the aged. Hence the available medical care is less productive (efficacious) in treating the elderly than in treating prime-age adults, which results in lower rates of utilization by the prime-age group.

Also unlike the situation in industrial countries is the fact that education does not seem to affect provider choice or the decision to seek formal care. The negligible effect of education most likely results from the small variation in education in the Ivorian sample. The average length of schooling is less than one year. Therefore, the estimated coefficient is probably not a true measure of the influence of education on utilization of medical care.

We find that males who experience an accident or illness are more likely to seek care, and in particular hospital care, than are females. This is again consistent with the theory that households will invest in their more productive members, or at least in the members who are considered to be more productive. It could also be a sign of gender bias that warrants more scrutiny than can be given in this study. Finally, the present Ivorian health care system may be more effective at treating the illnesses males generally experience than it is at treating the illnesses females generally experience.

The coefficients on the family structure variables indicate that individuals in households with fewer adults and more children are more likely to seek care from both hospitals and clinics. This is consistent with the hypothesis that having more adults in the household allows more time to better care for sick individuals at home, and having more children results in having less time to take care of the ill.

Finally, and not surprisingly, reductions in the severity of illness, as indicated by the number of healthy days, substantially reduce the probability of an adult seeking medical care, but it does not affect which alternative is chosen. This finding is common to almost all studies of utilization of medical care in both industrial and developing countries. One caveat is that the number of days an individual was healthy may be endogenous in a model of demand for medical care. To ensure the robustness of our price and income effects, we reestimated the model on samples of both adults and children without including the variable of healthy days. There was no difference in the estimated coefficients on the other variables.

The results from the model for children are similar to those for adults. The pattern of utilization of medical care through childhood is described by the coefficients on the age splines. They show that demand falls with age from zero to three years old and is flat thereafter. In other words, infants who experience an accident or illness are more likely to seek medical care than are older children and more likely to seek the higher-quality hospital care over clinic care.

As in the model for adults, the mother's education does not influence the choice of provider, and again this is attributed to the lack of variation in the data rather than interpreted as a true effect of education. Unlike the model for adults, however, the model for children shows no differences by sex. As in the adult model, severity of illness increases the demand for medical care, the number of adults in the household has a negative effect on the probability of going to both clinics and hospitals, and the number of children has a positive effect.

Price Elasticities

Since prices and income enter the demand functions in a highly nonlinear fashion, it is hard to assess the direction and magnitude of their effect on demand directly from the estimation results in table 6–2. To facilitate this, we estimate arc price elasticities of the demand for clinic and hospital care by income quartiles. The arc elasticities are obtained by sample enumeration (Train 1986) within each income quartile. More specifically, the probability of an individual choosing an alternative at the bottom and top of the specified price range is predicted for every individual in the income group. Only the price of the alternative being considered is changed for these calculations. To hold constant all characteristics except price and income, each individual was assigned other characteristics equal to the sample mean. Thus within an income group only the price varies, and within a price range only income varies. The arc price elasticity is then constructed by dividing the average percentage change in the sum of the probabilities by the average percentage change in the price. Thus an arc price elasticity of, say, −0.50 implies that a 10 percent increase in price will result in a 5 percent reduction in demand.

Arc price elasticities of the demand for clinic care and the demand for hospital care were calculated for three ranges of CFAF 50 each, ranging from free care to a fee of CFAF 150. These are within-sample calculations, since the opportunity cost of time averages about CFAF 100. The arc price elasticities are presented in tables 6–3 (for adults) and 6–4 (for children). Reading down a column of one of these tables

Table 6-3. Arc Price Elasticities for Adults in Rural Côte d'Ivoire

	Income quartile			
Fee[a]	*1*	*2*	*3*	*4*
Clinic				
0–50	−0.61	−0.58	−0.53	−0.38
50–100	−1.16	−1.03	−0.91	−0.56
100–150	−1.83	−1.71	−1.57	−0.93
Hospital				
0–50	−0.47	−0.44	−0.41	−0.29
50–100	−0.86	−0.81	−0.76	−0.51
100–150	−1.34	−1.27	−1.18	−0.71
Mean income[b]	33.28	64.44	99.52	222.87

Note: Quartile 1 is lowest.
a. Ivorian CFAFs.
b. Thousands of Ivorian CFAFs a month.

Table 6-4. Arc Price Elasticities for Children in Rural Côte d'Ivoire

	Income quartile			
Fee[a]	*1*	*2*	*3*	*4*
Clinic				
0–50	−0.90	−0.80	−0.67	−0.31
50–100	−1.81	−1.56	−1.29	−0.51
100–150	−2.82	−2.43	−1.98	−0.66
Hospital				
0–50	−0.65	−0.58	−0.49	−0.12
50–100	−1.34	−1.17	−0.98	−0.20
100–150	−2.32	−1.98	−1.60	−0.48
Mean income[b]	33.28	64.44	99.52	222.87

Note: Quartile 1 is lowest.
a. Ivorian CFAFs.
b. Thousands of Ivorian CFAFs a month.

shows the price elasticity moving down the demand curve, holding income constant. Reading across a row shows the change in the price elasticity as income rises, holding price constant.

The results show that the price elasticity of demand falls with income. Indeed, adults' and children's demand for both clinic and hospital care is more elastic at lower income levels than at the highest income levels. Both adults' and children's demand for clinic and hospital care in the bottom three quarters of the income distribution is in the price-elastic region, whereas the demand of those in the top income quartile is well into the inelastic region. In addition, children's demand for both clinic and hospital care is more price elastic than is adults' demand. The difference is smaller in the lower income groups but is substantial in the highest income group. These results indicate that user fees will be regressive in the sense that they reduce utilization of medical care by the poor substantially more than by the rich. Furthermore, user fees will reduce the utilization of medical care by children more than they will reduce utilization by adults. User fees can, however, generate substantial revenues without adverse effects on utilization in relatively better-off communities. These issues will be considered in chapter 7.

Implicit in the calculations of these price elasticities is the effect of travel time on utilization, working through the opportunity cost of time. To investigate the rationing effects of the location of facilities, we calculate travel time elasticities. To estimate how travel time affects demand across income groups, we need to allow wage rates (the opportunity cost of time) as well as income to vary across the income quartiles. We use the average agricultural wage rate associated with each income quartile for these calculations.

Arc travel time elasticities of the demand for clinic care and the demand for hospital care were calculated for four ranges of one hour each, covering zero to four hours. They are presented in tables 6–5 (for adults) and 6–6 (for children). Reading down a column of one of these tables reflects the change in the time elasticity for increasing travel time, holding income constant. Reading across a row reflects the change in the time elasticity as income rises, holding travel time constant.

The magnitude of the estimates of travel time elasticity is very similar to that of the estimates of price elasticity. This is not surprising since the opportunity cost of time is currently the whole price of medical care in Côte d'Ivoire; thus time prices ration the market. The estimates of elasticity show individuals in the bottom three fourths of the income distribution to be much more sensitive to the opportunity cost of time than richer individuals (those in the top quarter). Moreover, children's utilization of medical care is more sensitive to time than adults' utilization. One interesting result is that demand becomes slightly more time elastic as income rises over the bottom three income quartiles. This reflects the increase in wage rates (the opportunity cost of time) over these income groups.

These results imply that the opportunity cost of time is a bigger barrier to health care for poorer individuals than it is for richer

Table 6-5. Arc Travel Time Elasticities for Adults in Rural Côte d'Ivoire

Hours of travel time	Income quartile			
	1	2	3	4
Clinic				
0–1	−0.35	−0.32	−0.28	−0.14
1–2	−1.61	−0.57	−0.50	−0.24
2–3	−0.85	−0.83	−0.72	−0.33
3–4	−1.10	−1.09	−0.95	−0.42
Hospital				
0–1	−0.25	−0.23	−0.21	−0.11
1–2	−0.44	−0.42	−0.37	−0.19
2–3	−0.65	−0.62	−0.55	−0.27
3–4	−0.85	−0.84	−0.74	−0.34
Mean income[a]	33.28	64.44	99.52	222.87

Note: Quartile 1 is lowest.
a. Thousands of Ivorian CFAFS.

Table 6-6. Arc Travel Time Elasticities for Children in Rural Côte d'Ivoire

Hours of travel time	Income quartile			
	1	2	3	4
Clinic				
0–1	−0.53	−0.54	−0.54	−0.40
1–2	−0.93	−0.96	−0.98	−0.68
2–3	−1.33	−1.39	−1.43	−0.92
3–4	−1.72	−1.80	−1.88	−1.10
Hospital				
0–1	−0.41	−0.42	−0.42	−0.31
1–2	−0.71	−0.73	−0.75	−0.57
2–3	−1.03	−1.07	−1.12	−0.75
3–4	−1.37	−1.44	−1.52	−0.95
Mean income[a]	33.28	64.44	99.52	222.87

Note: Quartile 1 is lowest.
a. Thousands of Ivorian CFAFS.

individuals. Poorer individuals can less afford to lose productive time than can the rich. The lower income groups in our sample consist of subsistence farmers who obtain a good portion of their income in the form of self-produced food. Moreover, little income is available to purchase processed goods, which in turn implies that many hours must be spent in home production activities such as gathering wood and fetching water. Our results clearly underscore that poor people are not just money poor; they are also time poor. Therefore, increasing the supply of health care facilities in poor areas is a sine qua non for improving access. In other words, if improving the poor's access to medical care is a primary goal of social policy, providing the care free of charge is simply not enough.

Rural Peru

Since the data for Peru come from a survey instrument that is virtually identical to the one used for the Côte d'Ivoire survey, the empirical specification and the variables are constructed in almost the same way (table 6–7). Some differences are necessary because the institutional environment is different. Specifically, unlike Côte d'Ivoire, Peru has a large private health care sector that charges fees for utilization of its services. In this section we highlight the differences between Peru and Côte d'Ivoire that are relevant for estimating the Peruvian model of choice of provider.

Rural Peru has a mix of public and private medical care. The major provider of public medical care is the Ministry of Health, which operates hospitals and clinics. These institutions are administered at the health department (regional) level, where the user fee is set. In 1985–86 user fees were very low. We used the department's median clinic and hospital fee paid by individuals in our sample as monetary prices. There are fourteen departments in our sample. The total prices of clinic and hospital care are the sum of the department-level monetary prices and the opportunity cost of time, where the opportunity cost of time is calculated as the product of the round-trip travel time and the appropriate village-level agricultural wage rate. For children the opportunity cost of the mother's time is used. The dominant private providers are physicians. As was true in the case of Côte d'Ivoire, very few individuals reported seeking care from a traditional healer, so we leave them out of the analysis.

In the Peruvian specification, an individual experiencing an illness or accident has four alternatives: private doctor, government hospital, government clinic, or self-care. The distribution of provider choice in our sample is given in figure 6–2. Peruvians who experience an illness or injury use medical care only about half as much as Ivorians.

For each alternative, consumption net of expenditures on medical care is computed as income minus the sum of the monetary price of the alternative and the opportunity cost of travel time. Income is computed as the annual value of total household consumption divided by twelve, and the opportunity cost of time is the appropriate male or female wage rate times the round-trip travel time. The monetary price is the expected price of the initial consultation. It is constructed using the amount individuals reported paying for their initial consultation. For each alternative, we used the median reported payment in each village as the expected price of that provider. For each person in the village, this value is added to the individual's

Table 6-7. Descriptive Statistics for Rural Peru

Variable	Adults		Children	
	Mean	Standard deviation	Mean	Standard deviation
Clinic[a]	0.13	0.29	0.08	0.27
Hospital[a]	0.08	0.27	0.05	0.21
Doctor[a]	0.04	0.19	0.04	0.19
Clinic price[b]	1.32	0.76	1.37	0.86
Hospital price[b]	2.43	1.06	2.30	1.01
Doctor price[b]	22.27	16.57	23.95	16.59
Clinic travel time[c]	2.02	2.68	2.30	2.70
Hospital travel time[c]	4.56	6.23	4.83	6.11
Doctor travel time[c]	3.54	2.92	3.56	2.88
Monthly family income[b]	1,262.24	1,332.86	1,320.35	1,179.45
Hourly wage[b]	0.18	0.11	0.19	0.12
Age (years)	43.52	18.11	6.52	4.48
Male[a]	0.42	0.50	0.51	0.50
Education (years of schooling)	2.28	2.76	3.25	3.60
Healthy days in past four weeks	25.00	5.42	25.19	4.97
Number of adults in household	3.16	1.35	2.71	1.05
Number of children in household	2.62	2.01	3.83	1.59
Sample size	1,254		969	

a. Binary variable; equals one if alternative is chosen, zero otherwise.
b. June 1985 intis.
c. Round-trip travel time, reported in hours.

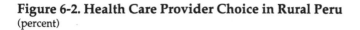

Figure 6-2. Health Care Provider Choice in Rural Peru
(percent)

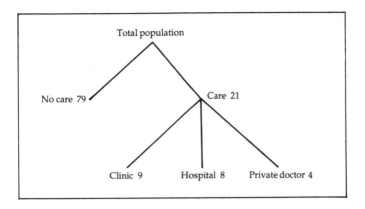

opportunity cost of travel time. On average, the monetary portion represents 82 percent of the total price.

The arguments of the alternative specific utility of quality functions are the same as used for Côte d'Ivoire. They are age, the number of healthy days last month, education, the number of other adults in the household, and the number of children in the household. Again, age is entered in spline form with the break occurring at forty years for adults and at three for children. Education is calculated as years of schooling, with mother's education being used for children.

In the Peruvian models, 37 percent of the households were excluded because they were in villages for which community-level information was unavailable. A few visits for obstetrics and other preventive purposes were also excluded. The final sample included 1,254 adults and 969 children under age 16 from 98 villages.

Thus the main differences between the Ivorian and the Peruvian models are that in Peru (1) the patient has four, rather than three, choices, and (2) the cost of obtaining care includes a monetary component as well as a travel time component. Note that for these rural samples Peruvian households are on average economically equivalent to their Ivorian counterparts: monthly per capita income is about $24 in Peru, $23 in Côte d'Ivoire.

Estimation Results

The results of maximum likelihood estimation of models for the choice of medical care provider for Peruvian children and adults are presented in table 6–8. As in the case of Côte d'Ivoire, the coefficients on the consumption term and its square are significantly different from zero in both adults' and children's models. These results confirm that the relative prices of the alternatives are important determinants

Table 6-8. NMNL Model of Provider Choice Estimates for Rural Peru

Variable	Adults		Children	
	Coefficient	t-statistic	Coefficient	t-statistic
Consumption[a]	5.13	2.14	6.88	2.37
Consumption squared[b]	−0.16	2.26	−0.21	2.04
Sigma	0.98	2.03	0.44	1.71
Private doctor				
Constant	−1.04	0.56	−2.30	1.99
Age 1[c]	0.01	0.40	−0.59	1.35
Age 2[d]	0.01	0.39	−0.15	1.84
Education	0.18	2.61	0.00	0.58
Male	−0.26	0.70	0.61	0.34
Children	0.03	0.31	0.27	1.91
Adults	−0.45	4.52	−0.83	2.36
Healthy days	−0.08	3.34	−0.26	3.30
Hospital				
Constant	1.61	1.63	3.12	1.15
Age 1[c]	0.06	3.48	−0.63	1.03
Age 2[d]	−0.02	1.47	0.02	0.42
Education	−0.20	4.51	0.06	0.25
Male	0.69	2.66	0.35	0.38
Children	0.09	1.46	−0.12	0.40
Adults	−0.19	2.59	−0.75	1.87
Healthy days	−0.11	6.31	−0.22	2.38
Clinic				
Constant	−1.65	1.91	3.58	1.39
Age 1[c]	0.03	1.65	−0.06	1.79
Age 2[d]	−0.01	0.45	0.02	0.42
Education	−0.10	2.25	0.12	1.97
Male	−0.03	0.13	0.43	0.96
Children	0.08	1.34	0.26	1.70
Adults	−0.06	0.66	−0.73	2.38
Healthy days	−0.06	3.64	−0.23	5.55
Sample size	1,254		913	
Log likelihood	−843		471	

NMNL = nested multinomial logit.
a. Variable divided by 100 for estimation.
b. Variable divided by 100,000 for estimation.
c. Adults age 16–40, children age zero to 3.
d. Adults over age 40, children over age 3.

of choice of provider. The direction and magnitude of the price and income effects are examined in the next section. This section discusses the effect of the other variables.

The estimated value of σ is 0.98 for adults and 0.44 for children. The estimate of σ in the adult model is significantly different from zero, but we could not reject the hypothesis that it is different from 1. Therefore, the adult model is consistent with utility maximization, but the MNL is not rejected in favor of the NMNL. The estimate of σ in the children's model is significantly different from zero and from 1. The children's model, therefore, is consistent with utility maximization and rejects the MNL specification in favor of the NMNL.

Utilization of medical care by Peruvian adults over the life span differs from the use of health care by adults in Côte d'Ivoire. The coefficients on the age splines indicate that an adult who experienced an accident or illness is progressively more likely to seek professional medical care as he or she gets older until he or she reaches the age of forty. After age forty, utilization remains constant.

Generally, we find that education strongly influences the decision to seek medical care and that more educated individuals choose the higher-quality options. This result conforms better to those from industrial countries than do the Ivorian results. The result strengthens the case that the negative effect of education on health care utilization for Côte d'Ivoire is attributable to the lack of variation in the education variable rather than to a true effect of education.

Females are much more likely to seek medical care to treat an illness or accident and are more likely to choose care in a hospital than care provided by a private physician or in a clinic. This is the opposite of the results for Côte d'Ivoire, but it is not clear whether this is a gender-bias effect or the result of rational decisions based on the expected productivity of the individual or on the efficacy of the health care system in treating gender-specific illnesses.

The other variables were commensurate with the Ivorian results. Not surprisingly, the higher the number of healthy days last month, the less likely is someone to seek medical care. The number of adults in the household has a negative effect on the probability of going to both clinics and hospitals, and the number of children has a positive effect. Thus families with more adults and fewer children are better able to care for sick family members at home than are families with fewer adults and more children.

The results from the model for Peruvian children are in general similar to those from the Peruvian adult model and conform to most studies on medical care demand in industrial countries. The age profile of utilization of health care is identical to that in Côte d'Ivoire.

Infants have the highest probability of seeking medical care to treat an accident or illness. The probability then falls with age until three years old and is flat thereafter, other things being equal.

We also found that more educated mothers are more likely to seek care in a clinic. This result is consistent with previous work. Although we are not aware of studies that focus exclusively on children's demand for health care in developing countries, mothers' education has been shown to have a strong positive effect on children's health status (see, for example, Strauss 1988). Utilization of medical care by Peruvian children does not differ by gender, which matches the results for Côte d'Ivoire.

Price Elasticities

To show the effect of prices (total costs) on utilization of medical care, we computed arc price and travel time elasticities. Arc price elasticities of the demand for the services of clinics, hospitals, and private doctors by income quartile are presented in tables 6–9 (for adults) and 6–10 (for children). The arc price elasticities are calculated for three fee levels, ranging from zero to 30 intis. Reading down a column of one of these tables shows the price elasticity moving down the demand curve, holding income constant. Reading across a row shows

Table 6-9. Arc Price Elasticities for Adults in Rural Peru

	Income quartile				
Fee[a]	1	2	3	4	Total
Private doctor					
0–10	−0.53	−0.36	−0.15	−0.00	−0.25
10–20	−0.91	−0.62	−0.25	−0.02	−0.38
20–30	−1.30	−0.87	−0.36	−0.03	−0.49
Hospital					
0–10	−0.57	−0.38	−0.16	−0.01	−0.26
10–20	−0.96	−0.64	−0.26	−0.02	0.39
20–30	−1.36	−0.91	−0.37	−0.04	−0.50
Clinic					
0–10	−0.31	−0.21	−0.08	−0.00	−0.15
10–20	−0.61	−0.40	−0.15	−0.01	−0.27
20–30	−0.95	−0.61	−0.23	−0.02	−0.39
Mean income[a]	395	783	1,267	2,620	1,286

Note: Quartile 1 is lowest.
a. June 1985 intis.

the change in the price elasticity as income rises, holding price constant.

The estimates show that the price elasticity of demand falls with income, so that poorer individuals are more price sensitive than are richer individuals. Indeed, the price elasticities, completely inelastic in the highest income quartile, enter the elastic range in the lowest income quartile in both the adults' and children's models. These estimates are commensurate with the results from the analysis of Côte d'Ivoire. They imply that user fees can be a significant source of income for the health care system. They also indicate that user fees will be regressive and may substantially reduce the use of medical care by the poor. Again, children's demand for clinic and hospital care is more price elastic than adult demand.

Note that the result that the price elasticity of demand falls with income implies that the willingness to pay for medical care increases with income. This result is very similar to one obtained by Birdsall and others (1983). Using a survey technique in which households in rural Mali were asked directly how much they would be willing to pay for improvements in health services and water supply, they found the income elasticity of the willingness to pay for these services to be around 0.35.

Arc travel time elasticities of the demand for the services of clinics, hospitals, and private doctors were calculated for four ranges of one

Table 6-10. Arc Price Elasticities for Children in Rural Peru

Fee[a]	Income quartile				
	1	2	3	4	Total
Private doctor					
0–10	−0.20	−0.16	−0.13	−0.06	−0.14
10–20	−0.44	−0.36	−0.27	−0.12	−0.29
20–30	−0.84	0.66	−0.48	−0.20	−0.52
Hospital					
0–10	−0.67	−0.48	−0.22	−0.03	−0.41
10–20	−1.18	−0.83	−0.38	−0.05	−0.64
20–30	−1.72	−1.20	−0.54	−0.09	−0.81
Clinic					
0–10	−0.76	−0.53	−0.24	−0.03	−0.46
10–20	−1.28	−0.89	−0.41	−0.06	−0.68
20–30	−1.80	−1.26	−0.57	−0.10	−0.83
Mean income[a]	395	783	1,267	2,620	1,286

Note: Quartile 1 is lowest.
a. June 1985 intis.

Table 6-11. Arc Travel Time Elasticities for Adults in Rural Peru

Hours of travel time	Income quartile				Total
	1	2	3	4	
Private doctor					
0–1	−0.04	−0.02	−0.01	−0.00	−0.02
1–2	−0.07	−0.04	−0.02	−0.01	−0.04
2–3	−0.09	−0.05	−0.04	−0.01	−0.05
3–4	−0.11	−0.07	−0.05	−0.02	−0.06
Hospital					
0–1	−0.03	−0.02	−0.01	−0.00	
1–2	−0.04	−0.03	−0.02	−0.00	−0.02
2–3	−0.06	−0.05	−0.03	−0.01	−0.04
3–4	−0.09	−0.06	−0.04	−0.01	−0.05
Clinic					
0–1	−0.03	−0.02	−0.01	−0.00	−0.02
1–2	−0.07	−0.04	−0.01	−0.00	−0.03
2–3	−0.08	−0.05	−0.02	−0.01	−0.04
3–4	−0.09	−0.06	−0.03	−0.01	−0.05
Mean income[a]	395	783	1,267	2,620	1,286

Note: Quartile 1 is lowest.
a. June 1985 intis.

Table 6-12. Arc Travel Time Elasticities for Children in Rural Peru

Hours of travel time	Income quartile				Total
	1	2	3	4	
Private doctor					
0–1	−0.04	−0.02	−0.01	−0.00	−0.02
1–2	−0.07	−0.04	−0.01	−0.00	−0.03
2–3	−0.10	−0.05	−0.02	−0.00	−0.04
3–4	−0.12	−0.06	−0.02	−0.00	−0.05
Hospital					
0–1	−0.04	−0.02	−0.01	−0.00	−0.02
1–2	−0.06	−0.03	−0.01	−0.00	−0.03
2–3	−0.09	−0.05	−0.02	−0.01	−0.04
3–4	−0.11	−0.06	−0.02	−0.01	−0.05
Clinic					
0–1	−0.03	−0.01	−0.01	−0.00	−0.01
1–2	−0.04	−0.02	−0.02	−0.00	−0.02
2–3	−0.06	−0.03	−0.02	−0.01	−0.03
3–4	−0.09	−0.04	−0.03	−0.01	−0.04
Mean income[a]	395	783	1,267	2,620	1,286

Note: Quartile 1 is lowest.
a. June 1985 intis.

hour each, covering zero to four hours. They are presented in tables 6–11 (for adults) and 6–12 (for children). The travel time elasticities are small relative to the price elasticities, which is unlike the Ivorian results. This is not surprising since the opportunity cost of time is a smaller portion of the total price of medical care in rural Peru. When monetary prices are large relative to the opportunity cost of time, the monetary prices ration the market and time prices are relatively unimportant. In Peru time costs are, on average, only 3 percent of the total private doctor price, 25 percent of the total hospital price, and 21 percent of the total clinic price. Therefore, we find much less reaction to changes in travel time than was the case in Côte d'Ivoire, where—in the absence of money prices—the total cost equals the opportunity cost of time lost in obtaining care.

Summary

Models of choice of medical care provider were estimated using data from the Living Standards Surveys of rural Côte d'Ivoire and rural Peru. The model for Côte d'Ivoire had government clinics and hospital care as alternatives; the model for Peru also included private doctor care. These specifications reflect the actual choices available to the population. In Côte d'Ivoire monetary prices were zero so that the market was rationed by the time costs involved in obtaining care from the providers. In Peru time costs were small relative to monetary prices. The models were estimated for children and adults separately. All models yielded similar price and income effects. The estimation results are overall consistent with economic theory.

Our primary purpose in estimating models of medical care provider choice is to evaluate the effect of charging user fees for government medical care. In evaluating the effect of user fees, cost recovery must be balanced against the potential effect on utilization. Indeed, one of the rationales for providing free care is to reduce barriers to access and increase utilization. This begs the question, Is the effect of user fees on utilization uniform across income groups? If poorer individuals' decisions to use medical care are more price elastic than richer individuals', user fees will be regressive in that they will reduce poorer individuals' utilization by more than that of richer individuals.

It is clear, then, that any evaluation of the proposal to institute user fees requires knowledge of the demand function from which price elasticities can be calculated. Price elasticities provide information about how user fees will affect utilization and revenues. Our estimates show that price is an important determinant of the decision to use medical care. In addition, we find that the price elasticity of demand falls in absolute value with income. More specifically, we find that demand is very elastic for individuals in the lowest income groups and quite inelastic for individuals in the highest income groups. These results are robust in that we observe them in the models for both Côte d'Ivoire and Peru and for both children and adults.

The results of our study, unlike those of most previous studies of the demand for medical care in developing countries, are quite consistent with current knowledge about the demand for medical care in industrial countries. The fact that we had access to high-quality data and used a model that solves some of the shortcomings in previous studies probably explains this.

Table 6-13. Reduced Form Model of Provider Choice in Rural Côte d'Ivoire

Variable	Adults		Children	
	Coefficient	t-statistic	Coefficient	t-statistic
Price	–6.121	5.16	–6.055	8.02
Clinic				
Constant	–0.284	0.54	0.813	2.06
Income	0.002	1.84	–0.002	1.83
Age 1[a]	0.012	0.09	–0.274	2.58
Age 2[b]	–0.031	3.34	0.024	0.83
Education	–0.020	0.48	0.003	0.66
Male	–0.106	–0.64	0.117	0.68
Children	0.040	1.48	0.057	1.98
Adults	–0.054	1.72	–0.110	2.48
Healthy days	–0.026	2.98	–0.024	2.02
Hospital				
Constant	0.096	0.16	0.653	1.43
Income	0.004	4.04	0.003	3.96
Age 1[a]	–0.010	0.62	–0.338	2.37
Age 2[b]	–0.042	3.93	0.014	0.38
Education	–0.028	0.57	–0.001	0.08
Male	0.053	2.48	–0.081	0.35
Children	0.040	1.31	0.082	2.23
Adults	–0.068	1.71	–0.126	2.86
Healthy days	–0.057	5.56	–0.050	3.30
Sample size	1,030		769	
Log likelihood	887.28		674.68	

a. Adults age 16–40, children age zero to 3.
b. Adults over age 40, children over age 3.

User fees have a great potential for cost recovery, but care must be taken in implementing them. Uniform user fees can generate substantial revenues but are very likely to reduce the utilization of medical care by the poor. Uniform user fees, then, would be regressive in that

Table 6-14. Reduced Form Model of Provider Choice in Rural Peru

Variable	Adults		Children	
	Coefficient	t-statistic	Coefficient	t-statistic
Price	−4.24	1.98	−8.39	2.25
Doctor				
Constant	−1.46	0.78	2.31	1.87
Income	0.19	1.21	0.35	1.81
Age 1[a]	0.01	0.40	−0.27	1.35
Age 2[b]	0.01	0.38	−0.13	1.77
Education	0.18	2.55	0.04	0.54
Male	−0.27	0.80	0.15	0.32
Children	−0.02	0.21	−0.26	1.86
Adults	0.45	4.29	0.47	2.34
Healthy days	−0.68	3.27	−0.10	3.26
Hospital				
Constant	−1.95	1.96	1.82	0.99
Income	0.21	3.37	0.22	1.62
Age 1[a]	0.06	3.58	−0.25	1.00
Age 2[b]	−0.02	1.48	0.02	0.31
Education	0.20	4.44	0.01	0.22
Male	−0.68	2.62	0.17	0.48
Children	0.07	1.19	−0.06	0.44
Adults	0.17	2.24	0.28	1.72
Healthy days	−0.11	6.20	−0.10	2.80
Clinic				
Constant	−1.80	2.08	1.04	1.19
Income	0.13	2.12	0.16	1.11
Age 1[a]	0.03	1.65	−0.27	1.72
Age 2[b]	−0.01	0.46	0.10	0.35
Education	0.10	2.16	0.07	1.90
Male	0.04	0.16	0.27	1.02
Children	0.02	1.19	−0.18	1.76
Adults	0.04	0.48	0.26	2.16
Healthy days	−0.05	3.61	−0.11	5.51
Sample size	1,254		913	
Log likelihood	830.83		469.08	

a. Adults age 16–40, children age zero to 3.
b. Adults over age 40, children over age 3.

they act as barriers to medical care for the poor but not for the members of the middle and higher income groups.

Note

1. An additional cost is the amount paid for transportation. In rural Côte d'Ivoire the vast majority of people reported walking, which suggests negligible transportation costs. Another potential time price is waiting and treatment time. These data are not available in the Living Standards Surveys.

Appendix

In this appendix we use the empirical specifications employed in earlier work on the demand for medical care in developing countries. The models were discussed in chapter 5. The purpose of this exercise is to provide results that are comparable to earlier work, even though, as we have argued, these specifications are inconsistent with utility maximization and therefore cannot be interpreted structurally. In these models, prices and income are entered linearly, and income has alternative specific coefficients. In conformity with other literature, the models are estimated as MNLs rather than as NMNLs. The data used to estimate alternative specific coefficients are described in chapter 6.

The results are presented in table 6–13 for Côte d'Ivoire and table 6–14 for Peru. It is interesting that statistically significant negative price effects are found in all four models. Moreover, income has a positive effect on the demand for health care and is statistically significant in most cases. These results suggest that problems with the data were probably a large part of the failure of some earlier studies to find significant price and income effects.

7

Options for Policy Reform

An assessment of the feasibility and desirability of introducing or raising user fees for medical care depends critically on consumers' responses to such a measure. More precisely, the potential for fees to generate revenue and the effect of fees on utilization and welfare depend on the price and income elasticities of demand. Reliable estimates of these elasticities are presented in this chapter.

Our results demonstrate that poorer people are much more sensitive to price changes than are the better off, so that price increases are likely to reduce the utilization of medical care by the poor more than that of the population as a whole. How then can these findings be used not only to judge whether user fees can be introduced to generate revenue but also to determine what fee levels can be set to prevent the poor from being cut off from obtaining medical care?

These questions are addressed by simulating the consequences of alternative price and reinvestment policies in various settings. For instance, the simulation evaluates the financial feasibility of locating a clinic in a poor remote village in the northern savannah area of Côte d'Ivoire. In the case of Peru, the evaluation considers, among other things, pricing policies for government clinics that take the private sector's price responses into account.

These simulations illustrate how, with the appropriate information, rational decisions can be based on the tradeoff between cost recovery and protecting the poor. To transform analytic results into recommendations about policy requires a comprehensive assessment of a country's political, cultural, and institutional conditions, including infrastructure, population trends, human resources planning, and fiscal realities. Policy therefore should be based on a much more comprehensive analysis than is presented in the following, and the simulations should be viewed as illustrations only and not as authoritative recommendations for the countries under study.

The analysis is limited to the tradeoff between cost recovery and access to health care. The feasibility and desirability of user fee policies are judged according to these criteria: (1) the potential for raising revenue, (2) the changes brought about in patterns of utilization of medical care, and (3) the effect on the welfare of the population, especially the poor. The first part of the chapter simulates policy scenarios for Côte d'Ivoire, the second for Peru.

All simulations are conducted by enumerating through the sample data. Two hypothetical villages are chosen from each country: one representing a population from the lowest quarter of the rural income distribution, the other the highest quarter. Observations corresponding to the hypothetical villages are selected from samples and used for the simulations. The simulations allow all relevant characteristics (such as education, family structure, and wage rate) as well as income to vary across the villages.

The model incorporates only the first visit to a provider. Since the model explains provider choice and not the total number of visits to a provider, the effect of user fees on follow-up visits cannot be simulated. Therefore, it must be assumed that the fee charged for the first visit covers the cost of treating the entire illness episode, regardless of the number of follow-up visits (in other words, it is tantamount to a registration fee customarily charged at clinics in developing countries).

Policy Options in Rural Côte d'Ivoire

The simulations presented in this section consider the consequences of alternative fee policies in two settings: a poor village in the northern savannah region and a wealthier village in the west forest region.

Rural Côte d'Ivoire can be divided into three regions: the northern savannah and the east and west forest. Of the three, the savannah is by far the poorest and the west forest the wealthiest. The simulations involve a savannah village whose residents would be in the lowest quarter of the rural income distribution in this area and a west forest village that is wealthier than average (in the highest quarter of the income distribution). Except for the consumption variables, the characteristics of these communities represent average villages in their region (see table 7–1).

Per capita consumption levels in 1985 in the relatively well-off west forest village (CFAF 156,000) were about two and a half times as large as in the poor savannah village (CFAF 60,000). The daily wage rate for agricultural workers in the west forest (CFAF 700) was more than twice the rate in the savannah (CFAF 300). Virtually all householders in the savannah are small farmers, three quarters of whom have fewer than five hectares of cultivable land. In comparison, three quarters of the farmers in the west forest have more than five hectares, and 25 percent have more than fifteen hectares.

The structure of agricultural production in the two regions is very different. The principal export crop in the savannah is cotton, which is grown by about one third of the farms. Most of the other agricultural production in the savannah consists of food for home consumption and for sale in the local markets. In contrast, the west forest is characterized by the cultivation of cocoa and coffee, which are the country's principal exports and sources of foreign exchange. More than 90 percent of the farms in the west forest cultivate cocoa or coffee.

The economy of both regions is only partially monetized; a large proportion of the food consumed is produced on household farms. Health care expenditures are likely to come from that part of the nonfood budget which consists of cash purchases and possibly from the monetized portion of the food budget. In the savannah, the share of food in total household consumption is about 70 percent, which leaves only CFAF 18,600 per capita for nonfood cash expenditures (table 7–1). Sixty percent of food consumption is home produced, which implies that an additional CFAF 16,560 cash per capita is spent on food. Thus in the savannah the total cash budget is CFAF 35,160 per capita, or about 60 percent of total consumption.

In the west forest much more money is available for cash expenditures. The share of food is about 60 percent of total consumption, which leaves about CFAF 62,400 per capita for nonfood cash expenditures, or about three and a half times what is available in the savannah. In addition, only 50 percent of the food budget is produced at home,

Table 7-1. Characteristics of West Forest and Savannah Villages, Côte d'Ivoire

Item	West Forest	Savannah
Daily agricultural wage (CFAF)	700	300
Per capita consumption (CFAF)	156,000	60,000
Per capita food consumption (CFAF)	93,600	41,400
Per capita nonfood consumption(CFAF)	62,400	18,600
Per capita cash expenditures (CFAF)	109,000	35,960
Percentage with piped water	85	79
Percentage with latrine or toilet facilities	44	20
Closest paved road (kilometers)	1	9
Closest medical professional (kilometers)	5	22
Percentage ill (past four weeks)	28	34
Percentage of ill who obtained medical care	45	37

which implies that CFAF 46,800 cash per capita is spent on food. Total cash expenditure in the west forest, then, amounts to about CFAF 109,000, or about three times the amount spent in the savannah.

The infrastructure and public health environment of a typical savannah village reflects the region's poverty. Approximately 21 percent of the households do not have access to relatively clean piped-in water and must obtain it from rivers, and 80 percent of the households have no latrine or toilet facilities. In contrast, only 15 percent of households in the west forest do not have access to clean water, and 56 percent do not have latrine or toilet facilities. The savannah is more isolated than the west forest: the closest paved road is located, on average, nine kilometers from savannah villages, whereas the closest paved road is less than one kilometer from west forest villages. Moreover, individuals in the savannah must travel an average of twenty-two kilometers to the nearest medical facility, whereas individuals in the west forest need to travel fewer than five kilometers on average.

The poor public health environment and poverty manifest themselves in the incidence of illness and utilization of medical care. In the four weeks preceding the survey, approximately 34 percent of individuals living in the savannah experienced an illness, whereas only 28 percent of those in the west forest experienced an illness. Of those who were ill, 37 percent consulted a medical professional in the savannah, and 45 percent consulted a professional in the west forest.

The variable cost of providing medical care in Côte d'Ivoire is useful in understanding the simulations. The variable cost of care can be used to evaluate the revenue-collecting potential of user fees in terms of costs recovered and in assessing the willingness to pay for improvements in the system relative to the cost of the improvements.

Clinics in rural Côte d'Ivoire are usually staffed with one nurse, whose salary is typically CFAF 115,000 a month. If a nurse were to spend between twenty and thirty minutes with each patient, he or she could see about 400 patients a month. Assuming this patient load, the average cost of labor per visit is CFAF 285. In addition to labor, an important variable cost is drugs, which amount to about CFAF 315 per visit (Barnum and Over 1989). Hence the average cost per visit is about CFAF 600. The assumption in this simulation is that the average variable cost of hospital care is the same as that of clinic care, although hospitals have substantially higher fixed costs.

User Fees without Reinvestment

As mentioned earlier, clinics and hospitals in Côte d'Ivoire do not charge user fees. To investigate how utilization of these facilities might change if the government instituted user fees, the following options are considered (see figures 7–1 and 7–2 for the results of the simulations):

Price scenario 1: setting hospital fees at CFAF 300
Price scenario 2: setting hospital fees at CFAF 600
Price scenario 3: setting clinic fees at CFAF 300 and hospital fees at CFAF 600
Price scenario 4: setting both clinic and hospital fees at CFAF 600.

These levels correspond with approximately half of the marginal cost (CFAF 300) and all of the marginal cost (CFAF 600). Thus if a clinic is operating at capacity (400 visits), these fees correspond with half cost recovery and full cost recovery.

The simulation begins with the base case, in which no fees are charged for either hospitals or clinics (the actual situation at present). In this case the opportunity cost of travel time rations the market. In the relatively well-off west forest village, where per capita income is higher and medical care facilities are closer, the use of medical care is substantially higher. Specifically, 45 percent of ill adults and 46 percent of ill children seek medical care, whereas in the poor savannah village only 33 percent of ill adults and 40 percent of ill children seek care.

The response of the two hypothetical villages to price increases differs dramatically. At a fee level representing full cost recovery for hospitals (scenario 2), the number of adults in the west forest seeking

Figure 7-1. User Fee Simulations for Adults in Côte d'Ivoire

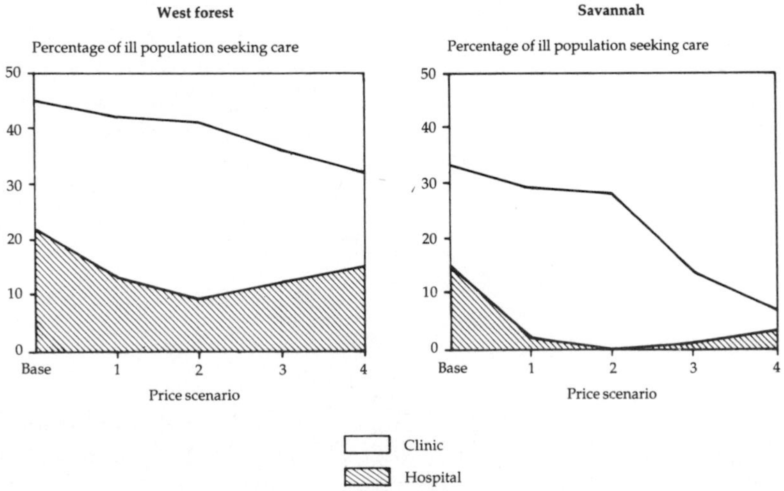

West forest

Percentage of ill population seeking care

Savannah

Percentage of ill population seeking care

Clinic
Hospital

care is about 41 percent, or a decline of about 9 percent. In the savannah village overall utilization falls below 30 percent, but the demand for hospital care is reduced to zero. Similar relative responses are observed for children. When fees are increased to the level of full cost recovery (CFAF 600) in clinics as well as in hospitals, both adults and children are effectively priced out of the market in the savannah; adults' utilization drops to 7 percent and children's to 3 percent. In the west forest 32 percent of adults and 15 percent of children still seek care.

One of the advantages of the nested multinomial logit specification is that it allows cross-price elasticities to differ across alternatives. Notice that as the hospital fee increases, most of those no longer choosing hospital care choose clinic care as opposed to self-care (figures 7–1 and 7–2). Therefore, user fees at hospitals can shift demand to clinics without substantially reducing total utilization.

Interestingly, at zero prices children's utilization rates are about the same as adults' in both the west forest and the savannah. Then, as prices rise, children's demand falls faster than adults' so that at prices representing full cost recovery children's utilization is lower than adults'.

The idea that a fee of CFAF 600 would generate enough revenue to cover the variable costs of clinic care relies on the assumption that there would be approximately 400 visits a month, that is, enough visits to cover one full-time nurse's salary plus the cost of drugs. For

Figure 7-2. User Fee Simulations for Children in Côte d'Ivoire

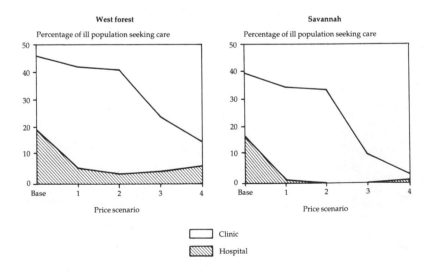

planning purposes it is important to take into account the aggregate demand response to determine if there would be sufficient utilization. The question, then, is what size communities will support clinics at the various levels of cost recovery. From the information on the probabilities of seeking care and of experiencing an illness (see table 7–1) we can derive the approximate population necessary to generate 400 visits to a clinic at the three fee levels of zero cost recovery, half cost recovery, and full cost recovery (see table 7–2). These estimates were derived under the assumption that hospitals charged a user fee of CFAF 600.

At zero cost recovery a population of about 1,750 in the west forest and about 3,650 in the savannah would fully utilize a clinic. At fee levels that would cover about half of costs the population necessary to support a clinic in the savannah is about four times the size of that in the west forest, and for full cost recovery the savannah population has to be seven times larger. The sizable variation in the population necessary to support a clinic reflects the dramatic differences in utilization rates in the two regions at fee levels of CFAF 300 and CFAF 600.

Table 7–2 presents estimates of the population necessary to support a clinic in a village under the various user fee scenarios. If the population necessary to support a clinic does not live in a village but is distributed over a larger area, travel costs would be higher and utilization rates lower than those implicit in table 7–2. Consequently, the results understate the size of population necessary to support a clinic in an area where population is not very dense.

User Fees with Reinvestment

When monetary prices are low the opportunity cost of time rations the demand for health care. Typically, medical care facilities are located much closer to patients in wealthier regions (urban areas) than in poorer regions (rural areas). In rural Côte d'Ivoire, individuals living in the west forest travel on average less than a half hour one

Table 7-2. **Population Necessary to Support a Clinic in Côte d'Ivoire**

Price scenario	West Forest	Savannah
2 (zero cost recovery)	1,750	3,650
3 (half cost recovery)	1,900	8,100
4 (full cost recovery)	2,850	20,300

way to a clinic, whereas savannah residents must travel more than one and a half hours on average. Thus a uniform schedule of fees implies a regressive pricing policy even at zero monetary cost.

This section presents an evaluation of the effect on consumers' welfare of the proposal to locate clinics in villages that lack facilities and then charge user fees for access. The net benefit to individuals of such a policy depends on whether the reduction in welfare—having to pay user fees—is less than the improvement in welfare—having access to medical care facilities in the village. The welfare-neutral fee is the amount consumers would be willing to pay not to have to travel (that is, the compensating variation). If the welfare-neutral fee is more than the marginal cost of medical care, the policy improves welfare. If the welfare-neutral fee is less than the marginal cost, the policy reduces welfare.

The welfare-neutral prices are derived from experiments with compensating variations. Three welfare-neutral prices are calculated for an average individual in each of the two hypothetical villages: how much an individual is willing to pay not to have to travel to free clinics that are at present one hour away, two hours away, and three hours away. The experiments are conducted assuming that the closest hospital is four hours away and charges a user fee of CFAF 600.

The welfare-neutral prices are reported in table 7–3. Reading across a row shows the change in willingness to pay in relation to the distance to the clinic. The welfare-neutral prices increase with this distance for both children and adults in both villages. West forest residents are willing to pay about three times as much as adults in the savannah. These welfare-neutral fees are 5 percent and 15 percent of the average cost of providing clinic care. Hence, implementing the proposal to locate clinics in villages and charge users average costs at the new and old facilities will lead to a reduction in welfare. For the policy to be welfare improving, a subsidy of approximately 90 percent is required. Before drawing the most important conclusions about

Table 7-3. Willingness to Pay for Reduced Travel Time in Côte d'Ivoire
(CFAF)

	Travel time to clinic		
Group	*One hour*	*Two hours*	*Three hours*
West forest adults	46	62	78
Savannah adults	16	22	27
West forest children	28	46	57
Savannah children	14	19	38

policy from these results, we will simulate the outcome of a similar set of policy alternatives for two hypothetical villages in Peru.

Policy Options in Rural Peru

Peru can be divided into three large regions: the forest, the sierra, and the coast. Of the three the sierra is by far the poorest and the coast the richest. Residents of the sierra, among the poorest in the world, have incomes similar to those of residents of the poorest regions in Côte d'Ivoire. Residents of the coast are quite well off and indeed are much wealthier than residents of the west forest region in Côte d'Ivoire. This section presents simulations of the likely effects of various user fee policies in two hypothetical villages: a poor village in the sierra whose residents are in the lowest quarter of the rural Peruvian income distribution, and a wealthy village on the coast whose residents are in the highest quarter of rural income distribution.

The characteristics of these two villages are presented in table 7–4. The differences in wealth are apparent. Average agricultural workers' daily wage rates on the coast are twice those in the sierra, and per capita annual consumption on the coast (2,520 intis) is approximately two and a half times that in the sierra (960 intis). In the poorer sierra, about 76 percent of total consumption is spent on food, which leaves only 230 intis per capita for other purposes. On the coast, only 60 percent of total consumption is spent on food, or—in absolute value— more than three times what is spent in the sierra.

The infrastructure and public health conditions also reflect the poverty of the sierra. Only 10 percent of households in the sierra have access to relatively clean piped water, and the rest must obtain it from rivers and streams. On the coast, 59 percent of households have piped

Table 7-4. Characteristics of Sierra and Coastal Villages, Peru

Item	Sierra	Coast
Daily agricultural wage (intis)	1.3	2.6
Per capita consumption (intis)	960	2,520
Per capita food consumption (intis)	730	1,590
Per capita nonfood consumption (intis)	230	930
Percentage with piped water	10	59
Percentage with latrine or toilet facilities	31	41
Closest medical professional (hours)	4	1.25
Percentage ill (past four weeks)	43	30
Percentage of ill who obtained medical care	24	30

water. Only 31 percent of sierra households have latrine or toilet facilities, whereas 41 percent have these facilities in the coastal area. Moreover, the closest medical facility is four hours' travel time on average from sierra households and only one and a quarter hours from coastal households.

These differences manifest themselves in morbidity rates and in the utilization of health care. In the sierra, approximately 43 percent of all individuals experienced an illness in the four weeks before the survey, and 24 percent of them sought formal medical attention. Thirty percent of coastal residents experienced an illness, and 30 percent of them sought formal medical attention.

As for the recurrent costs of medical care, data from the Peru Living Standards Survey indicate that a nurse's monthly salary is about 1,000 intis on average. If approximately 400 visits a month are assumed, the average labor cost per visit is about 2.5 intis. The cost of drugs for respiratory and digestive problems averages 15 intis an illness (Gereffi 1988). This amounts to an average cost of about 17.5 intis a visit.

User Fees without Reinvestment

Government clinics and hospitals at present charge small user fees of 1 to 5 intis depending on the region. This section concerns the likely effects of increasing user fees to levels representing half and full cost recovery. Unlike Côte d'Ivoire, Peru has a large private sector. Increases in prices at government facilities are likely to shift demand to the private sector. The increased demand may cause private doctors to increase their prices and consequently further reduce the number of ill individuals who obtain medical care. Thus a complete evaluation of user fees must take into account the private doctor supply response. One difficulty is that there is no information about the slope of the private doctor supply function. Therefore, two extreme scenarios are used in the belief that the likely scenario is somewhere in between. The two scenarios are that there is no price response among private doctors and that there is an increase in prices charged by private doctors equal to the increase in fees at public facilities.

The simulation considers first the effect of charging user fees at hospitals and then the effect of extending fees to clinics. Fee levels representing half and full cost recovery are considered. In the base case clinics and hospitals charge zero fees. It is important to note, however, that this is not the actual situation, since government facilities charge small fees. The user fee simulations involve the following options:

Price scenario 1: setting hospital fees at 7.5 intis

Price scenario 2: setting hospital fees at 15 intis

Price scenario 3: setting clinic fees at 7.5 intis and hospital fees at 15 intis

Price scenario 4: setting both clinic and hospital fees at 15 intis.

These simulations are performed twice. The first set assumes that the private sector does not respond at all to changes in the price of public health services. The second set assumes that private doctors raise their prices by an amount equal to the increase in fees at public facilities. The results of the simulations are reported in figures 7–3 and 7–4, which show the percentage of the ill population that obtains medical care from each of the available alternative providers, including self-care, under each of the four price scenarios.

In the base case, in which hospitals and clinics charge no fees, 29 percent of adults and children from the relatively well-off coast obtain professional medical care to treat an accident or illness. In the poorer sierra village, 27 percent of adults and 24 percent of children seek professional medical care.

As was the case for Côte d'Ivoire, an increase in user fees affects utilization of health care in dramatically different ways in the two villages. The figures show that charging user fees that represent full cost recovery at both hospitals and clinics has a negligible effect on the utilization of professional medical care by both adults and children from the coastal village. Raising user fees in the sierra clinics and hospitals does have a significant effect on utilization. If it is assumed that private doctors do not raise their prices in response to an increase in fees at public facilities, an increase in hospital fees in the sierra to the level of full cost recovery (price scenario 2), reduces adults' demand for hospital services by about 42 percent and children's by about 76 percent. Total utilization of medical care by adults falls by about 6 percent, and total utilization by children falls by about 16 percent. An additional increase in clinic fees to the level of full cost recovery (price scenario 4) reduces adults' demand for clinic services by 39 percent and children's by 62 percent. Moreover, with fees at the level of full cost recovery, adults' total demand falls by 24 percent and children's by 38 percent. If it is assumed that private doctors raise their prices by an amount equal to the increase in fees at public facilities, the reduction in total utilization is even larger. With fees at the level of full cost recovery (price scenario 4), adults' total demand is reduced by 44 percent and children's by 46 percent.

For a clinic to be financially self-sufficient (apart from capital costs), it is assumed that there must be 400 visits a month. Table 7–5 reports the population necessary to generate this number of visits under three of the price scenarios. The population base needed in the sierra is smaller than that on the coast under price scenarios 2 and 3 because the probability of developing an illness is greater in the sierra than on the coast. The population bases needed under the price scenarios

Figure 7-3. User Fee Simulations for Adults in Peru

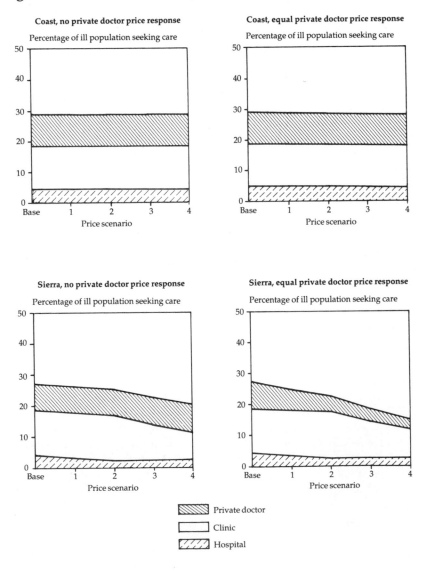

representing lower cost recovery are larger than in Côte d'Ivoire because both the probability of illness and the rate of utilization are higher in Côte d'Ivoire than in Peru.

Figure 7-4. User Fee Simulations for Children in Peru

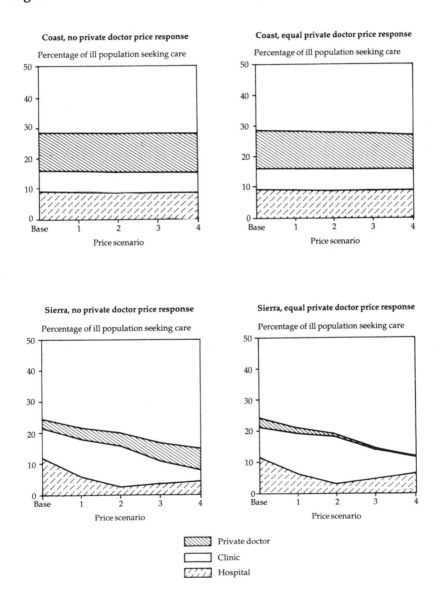

User Fees with Reinvestment

Is it feasible to improve access to health care by opening new clinics (thereby reducing travel time) and charging users the recurrent cost of operating the new facilities? Investigating this question is a prerequisite to evaluating whether increased access to medical care can be self-financed by users. The answer to the question is derived by calculating welfare-neutral fees, which are the prices people are willing to pay to avoid traveling long distances to obtain medical care. Recall that the willingness to pay is calculated as a compensating variation using the formulas derived in chapter 6. Three welfare-neutral prices are calculated for an average individual in both hypothetical villages: the amount an individual is willing to pay not to have to travel one hour, two hours, and three hours to a clinic. The experiments are conducted assuming that the closest hospital is four hours away and charges a user fee of 15 intis, and a private doctor is two hours away and charges 20 intis.

The welfare-neutral prices are reported in table 7–6. Reading across a row indicates the change in the welfare-neutral price as the travel time rises. Residents of the sierra village are willing to pay almost nothing to avoid traveling, whereas residents of the coastal village are willing to pay about 10 percent of the recurrent costs of operating a clinic.

Table 7-5. Population Necessary to Support a Clinic in Peru, by Degree of Private Doctor Price Response

Price scenario	Coast		Sierra	
	None	*Equal*	*None*	*Equal*
2 (zero cost recovery)	17,400	17,100	9,600	8,800
3 (half cost recovery)	18,100	17,300	15,000	12,700
4 (full cost recovery)	18,400	17,300	26,200	20,300

Table 7-6. Willingness to Pay for Reduced Travel Time in Peru
(intis)

Group	Travel time to clinic		
	One hour	*Two hours*	*Three hours*
Coastal adults	0.56	1.07	1.54
Sierra adults	0.00	0.01	0.02
Coastal children	1.01	1.94	2.80
Sierra children	0.03	0.06	0.09

Implications for Policy

The estimated demand functions defined earlier were used in this chapter to simulate the likely effect of various user fee policies in two hypothetical villages in each of the two countries under study: one poor village and the other richer. Although the countries are very different, the simulation results are quite similar. The results indicate that user fees at the levels of half and full marginal cost recovery would effectively price residents of the poorer communities out of the medical care market. Alternatively, user fees at these levels do not seem to substantially deter medical care utilization by residents of the wealthier villages. Thus it appears that user fees are a potential source of substantial revenue for the health care sector, but poorer communities need to be protected from the adverse effect of substantial fees on utilization.

Two other results of the simulations have immediate implications for policy. First, charging fees for higher levels of care (hospitals, for example) generally causes individuals to switch to other types of care rather than to drop out of the medical care market. Second, user fees seem to have a greater negative effect on children's utilization of medical care than on adults'.

The results of simulations in which facilities charge fees at the level of full cost recovery and travel time is reduced to zero show that this policy would substantially reduce welfare and utilization in both richer and poorer villages. Hence this extreme expansion of the health care system in rural areas cannot be completely user financed and requires about a 90 percent subsidy to be welfare improving.

It is important to place these results in the context of the family budget. Given the probability of experiencing an illness, the probability of seeking medical care, and the cost of care, we can derive the subsidy provided to an individual when medical care is provided free of charge. Zero user fees imply an annual subsidy of about CFAF 1,460 per capita in the wealthier Ivorian village and CFAF 960 per capita in the poorer village. The subsidy amounts to 0.9 percent of the total budget for wealthy families and about 1.6 percent of the total budget for poorer families. Since medical care is likely to be purchased at the expense of nonfood items, the budget shares become even larger. The subsidies amount to 2.3 percent of nonfood expenditures for wealthy families and 5.2 percent for poorer families.

For Peru, the annual per capita subsidy to residents of wealthier villages such as the hypothetical coastal one is 30 intis, whereas the subsidy to residents of poor villages such as the one in the sierra is 43 intis. This amounts to 1.2 percent of total consumption for the wealthier family and 4.5 percent of total consumption for the poor family, or 3.2 percent of the nonfood budget for the wealthy family and about 18.7 percent for the poor. The results can be summarized by pointing out that people are willing to pay 2 to 3 percent of their nonfood budget for medical care but are not willing to pay 5 percent or more.

8
Conclusion

The main analytical result of this study is that the demand for medical care is responsive to changes in price. Moreover, the price elasticity of demand falls as income rises. The result that demand is price responsive is in accordance with most of the literature on industrial countries as well as with a few recent studies on the developing world (Cretin and others 1988, Alderman and Gertler 1988, and Mwabu 1988) but differs with a few of the other studies on the demand for medical care in developing countries. Indeed, a review of this early evidence on price responsiveness led to the conclusion that prices are not relevant in the decision to seek medical care (World Bank 1987). The review of the literature in chapter 5 presented various reasons for this surprising and—given the evidence available from industrial countries—paradoxical finding.

All studies mentioned, including our own, draw their conclusions from the statistical analysis of cross-sectional sample data. Based on the behavior of households and individuals who currently face different prices and other costs of access, demand equations are postulated and estimated and the coefficient for the price effect is statistically tested against the null hypothesis of a zero price effect. Ideally, experiments would be conducted in which alternative price regimes are implemented and utilization patterns before and after the change are compared. Given the straightforwardness of this concept, the lack of such experiments is surprising. In fact, we found just one study that reports on such a before-and-after evaluation.

Enyimayew (1988) reports results from the Ashanti-Akim experience in Ghana. After the introduction of user fees in 1985, attendance dropped to one quarter of the previous level. In the larger urban-based health stations attendance recovered quickly, but two and a half years after the introduction of user fees, small rural-based stations that serve primarily the poor see only a fraction of the patients they saw before and operate at less than half of their optimal level. This result is strikingly similar to the simulation results presented in chapter 7: user fees can be introduced in relatively well-off regions without significantly affecting utilization of health care, but user fees will constitute an effective barrier to medical care for the poor.

Other corroborating evidence for our analytical findings is more anecdotal. For instance, Dunlop (1987) reports that in Ethiopia revenues for outpatient care actually decreased after a fee increase was implemented, which implies that the price elasticity of demand exceeds –1.0 in absolute value. The same study, however, also reports arc price elasticities of between –0.05 and –0.50, so the evidence is mixed, except for the fact that demand is sensitive to prices. Boa (1987) reports that about half of the ill peasants in Hubei province, China, who do not obtain medical care report the high price as the major deterrent. Two thirds of the poor in the mountainous areas say they do not seek care because the price is too high.

In sum, we are quite confident that our main findings are correct and should be taken seriously by those who propose to charge user fees as a means of generating revenue for the delivery of health care. The end of this chapter presents a summary of the implications for policy of our findings. But first we will draw attention to some of the shortcomings of our study and thus, among other things, sketch an agenda for future research.

Suggestions for Future Research

To improve the understanding of the determinants of demand for medical care, the model used in this book should be employed in a more detailed investigation of the determinants of more specific aspects of health care utilization. The extension is necessary since the present analysis was restricted to the choice of provider. It is a straightforward matter to include in the model the total number of visits as well as outlays for follow-up consultations. The total cost of access, including, for instance, out-of-pocket transportation costs, would ideally be more precise. The data required for such a change in the model are extensive, but a carefully prepared household survey focusing on health and the utilization of medical care could incorporate questions to obtain such information.

It will be somewhat more difficult—but not less important—to become more specific about exactly what is meant by the demand for medical care. For instance, the willingness to pay for preventive care is probably quite different from the willingness to pay for curative care. The price elasticity of drugs and the demand for care for chronic diseases will differ from those for acute care, emergency care, and maternal and child health care. This study focuses on the demand for acute primary outpatient care. Subsequent research should focus on other specific types of medical care. This endeavor, by itself, does not cause any conceptual difficulties. It does imply, though, that much more attention needs to be paid to the measurement of health status. Self-reported health status (days of normal activity lost because of an illness or injury) is likely to contain insufficient information if one is interested in explaining the choice between, say, visiting a midwife or a hospital emergency clinic.

Others (for example, Strauss 1988) would argue that health status should be treated as endogenous. Although this is theoretically correct, there was no effect on the estimation results in this study when endogenous measures of health status were removed. Again, this issue may become very difficult to deal with empirically if demand equations specific to a certain kind of health care are being estimated using measures of health status specific to certain illnesses. This analysis requires a longitudinal design in which patients are followed over time so that specific investments (use of medical care) can be evaluated for their effect on future improvements in health.

This book does not address certain aspects of health care financing through user fees. These areas deserve to be accorded high priority by researchers on health economics.

First, researchers should consider the effect of the quality of care (for example, the amount of training received by the doctor or the availability of drugs and diagnostic equipment) on the demand for care. The demand equation may shift if the quality of the services provided increases. If such a shift is large enough, it may offset the negative effect on utilization of an increase in the price of care. This is an empirical question that can and should be researched using provider-specific data in conjunction with data from household surveys.

Second, the responses of the private sector to pricing policies in the public health care sector should be studied. As demonstrated in the policy simulations for Peru, potential revenues for the public sector may carry over to the private sector if fees for government clinics are raised. Although this is not necessarily a negative development (it could, for instance, free an overburdened public sector to provide more care to the poor), it might have significant consequences for the amount of revenue raised. A better understanding of supply responses in the private health care sector (will the private sector increase its price in response to the increase in demand, or will it expand its facilities, or both?) is necessary to make a more complete judgment about the feasibility of financing medical care through user fees.

Third, much more work can be done to better target public health care facilities to benefit the poor. Even in a relatively small country such as Côte d'Ivoire, regional differences in levels of welfare are significant. Given our simulation results, it makes sense to subsidize medical care in such areas as the savannah in Côte d'Ivoire and the sierra in Peru. At the same time, user fees can be introduced in the better-off areas without large negative effects on utilization. If welfare differences are very large, some form of cross-regional subsidization may be a desirable and feasible option.

Fourth, analytical work should be carried out on how to protect the poor by providing them with health insurance. Little work is being done in this area because targeting the poor is very difficult without a reliable system for reporting income, and these systems do not exist in many developing countries. But, for example, in countries where governments have created a monopoly on export crops grown by small farmers, a tiny percentage of the revenue from these crops could be earmarked for providing health insurance to these farmers. Such a plan could benefit cotton growers in Côte d'Ivoire, for example, who are a large fraction of the poor. Alternatively, just as subsidies for the delivery of health care can vary by region, so can subsidies for health insurance vary by region or even by village, if they were based, say, on production of export crops. Clearly, the ramifications of such policies need to be worked out, but the examples suggest that there are many alternatives to the customary across-the-board subsidy schemes that, in practice, always turn out to be regressive. More analytical work in this area is needed, as well as more innovative real-world experimentation.

Finally, more work needs to be done on the effect of utilization of medical care on health. We take as given the assumption—and it is a significant one—that medical care improves health and that patients' willingness to pay reflects their knowledge of and the value of the health benefits. Research in this area will help to identify externalities and social benefits beyond what patients are willing to pay. Under-standing the efficacy of medical care in developing countries is critical for the prudent and cost-effective expansion of the health care system.

Suggestions for Implementation of Policies

The four most important empirical findings of this study are:

- The demand for medical care is price sensitive.
- The poor are more price sensitive than the rich.
- Care for children is more price elastic than care for adults.

- An increase in the price of one provider is more likely to lead patients to turn to another provider than to opt for self-care.

How, then, can user fees be implemented and the poor protected at the same time? Do these results imply that user fees should not be introduced as a source of revenue for the health care sector? Not at all. Demand overall is price inelastic with an order of magnitude of about −0.2 to −0.4, which implies that increases in prices will raise substantial revenue. In addition, there are many good reasons other than resource mobilization for reintroducing price signals to the health care system (see, for example, World Bank 1987). What the results imply is that just as providing medical care free of charge to the entire population is a regressive and unattainable policy, so will the across-the-board introduction of user fees be regressive and—in poor areas—unattainable.

The first result, that the demand for medical care is responsive to price changes, has straightforward implications for the potential for collecting revenue: since the demand for medical care will fall if prices rise, revenues will be lower than without a price response. This is particularly the case if there are close substitutes for public facilities, such as private care.

The second result, that the poor are more price sensitive than the rich, implies that the potential for collecting revenue in poor areas is very low. Clinics in poor areas cannot survive financially unless they are heavily subsidized. The poor's willingness to pay for medical care is so low that they are effectively being priced out of the market even by fees that are just a fraction of marginal costs. Our results indicate that fees can be charged without a significant drop in utilization if the cost of medical care takes no more than 2 to 3 percent of the household's nonfood budget. Though we are hesitant to prescribe this number as a rule of thumb, it does suggest that the estimated budget share for medical care can give a first indication about the feasible level of user fees. The practical implication of these results is that uniform user fees are regressive and that some sort of price discrimination is necessary to simultaneously achieve the goals of cost recovery and equity. In countries without good systems for reporting income, targeting the poor for price discounts is administratively difficult. One immediate alternative is geographic price discrimination: charge lower prices at facilities that primarily serve low-income regions. In addition, policymakers may want to opt for the gradual introduction of user fees, starting at a level that will result in expenditures of no more than about 2 percent of the household nonfood budget. Careful evaluation of the changes in patterns of utilization resulting from such charges should provide guidance for subsequent policies regarding the fee levels. Of course, such an approach implies that fees in poorer areas have to be set well below those in better-off regions.

If our third result, that care for children is more price sensitive than care for adults, holds up to scrutiny, it too contains a strong warning against an across-the-board introduction of user fees. Clearly, it would be penny wise and pound foolish for a developing country not to invest in the health of its younger generation. With the formation of human capital being one of the driving forces of economic development, there is much to be said for providing medical care to children who need it. It would be logistically simple to exempt care for children from increases in the fee structure for medical care or at least to differentiate between fees for children's and adults' health care. An argument based on humanitarian motives would probably make such a differentiation politically feasible. If our results turn out to be generally true, such a policy would also make good economic sense.

The fourth result, that an increase in the price of one provider is more likely to lead patients to turn to another provider than to opt for self-care, provides another argument in favor of a differentiated introduction of user fees in the health care system. The result suggests that fees should be introduced or increased for higher levels of care (say, at hospitals). If, on the one hand, after the implementation of such a policy, the demand for hospital care decreases significantly while the demand for clinic care increases, any increase in the charge for clinic care is likely to result in an overall reduction of medical care utilization. If, on the other hand, the demand response to the hospital fee is modest, the government could experiment with a gradual introduction of fees in the lower echelons of the health care system.

The overall message to policymakers is thus one of gradation and differentiation. The best policy advice will be derived from carefully monitoring the effect of real-world experiments. The selective introduction of modest fees, followed by a careful evaluation of the resulting changes in patterns of health care utilization, will guide subsequent policy measures and corrective actions.

Health is vital in the development process. The existing health care infrastructure is in poor condition, and more financial resources are needed to improve the situation. Given the current economic climate and the tight fiscal policies many developing countries have to follow to return to a path of sustained economic growth, additional financing is unlikely to come from government resources. Are user fees the answer? This study has shown that, in general, user fees can generate significant revenue if introduced carefully. The best policy is likely to be one that starts with charging modest fees for higher-level care. Fees approaching the marginal cost of care, however, will effectively cut the poor out of the health care market. Thus large subsidies continue to be necessary to provide medical care to the poor.

This book has not addressed the question of how much governments should spend on medical care regardless of whether it is financed with general tax revenue or with user fees. Rather, it has been concerned with what consumers are willing to pay for improvements in the health care system. If consumers are not willing to pay for such improvements, then the question remains, Should society be willing to pay and how much? As discussed in chapter 2, the rationale for public investment is that human capital and therefore productivity and positive health-related externalities should be improved. Thus what society is willing to pay depends on the amount of health the marginal investment in medical care produces and the size of the health-related externalities. It is well beyond the scope of this study to answer these questions and indeed inappropriate to decide the extent to which governments should subsidize the provision of medical care beyond what consumers are willing to pay. It is hoped that this book has contributed to the base of knowledge necessary for governments to make their own decisions about investment.

In the past many countries have opted to eliminate all financial barriers to obtaining medical care. This has led to a resource-starved health care system in which the limited supply of services is rationed by nonprice mechanisms. In spite of good intentions, the result is a highly inequitable, regressive distribution of public health services. User fees can significantly increase the resources available for improving the health care system. If these fees are introduced in a differentiated way, the policy can generate revenues and improve the equity of the system. If, however, no special measures are taken, user fees will perpetuate the inequitable distribution of health care in the developing world.

References

The word "processed" describes works that are reproduced from typescript by mimeograph, xerography, or similar means; such works may not be cataloged or commonly available through libraries, or may be subject to restricted circulation.

Acton, J. P. 1975. "Nonmonetary Factors in the Demand for Medical Service: Some Empirical Evidence." *Journal of Political Economy* 83:595–614.

Akin, John S., C. Griffin, D. K. Guilkey, and B. M. Popkin. 1984. *The Demand for Primary Health Care in the Third World*. Totowa, N.J.: Littlefield, Adams.

———. 1986. "The Demand for Primary Health Care Services in the Bicol Region of the Philippines." *Economic Development and Cultural Change* 34, no. 4 (July): 755–82.

Alderman, Harold, and Paul Gertler. 1988. "The Substitutability of Public and Private Medical Care Providers for the Treatment of Children's Illnesses in Urban Pakistan." International Food Policy Research Institute, Washington, D.C. Processed.

Arrow, K. J. 1963. "Uncertainty and the Welfare Economics of Medical Care." *American Economic Review* 53:941–73.

Balassa, Bela. 1985. "Public Finance and Social Policy—Explanation of Trends and Developments: The Case of Developing Countries." In Guy Terny and A. J. Culyer, eds., *Public Finance and Social Policy: Proceedings of the 39th Congress of the International Institute of Public Finance, Budapest, 1983*. Detroit: Wayne State University Press.

Barnum, H., and Mead Over. 1989. "Planning for the Recurrent Cost of the Health Sector: An Application to Côte d'Ivoire." World Bank, Population and Human Resources Department, Washington, D.C. Processed.

Barrera, Albino. 1987. "Maternal Schooling and Child Health." Ph.D. diss., Yale University, New Haven, Conn. Processed.

————. 1990. "The Role of Maternal Schooling and Its Interaction with Public Health Programs in Child Health Production." *Journal of Development Economics* 32 (January): 69–91.

Baumol, William J., and David F. Bradford. 1970. "Optimal Departures from Marginal Cost Pricing." *American Economic Review* 60:265–83.

Becker, Gary. 1965. "A Theory of the Allocation of Time." *Economic Journal* 75, no. 299: 493–517.

Behrman, Jere R. 1988. "The Impact of Economic Adjustment Programs on Health and Nutrition in Developing Countries." In David E. Bell and Michael R. Reich, eds., *Health, Nutrition, and Economic Crises: Approaches to Policy in the Third World*. Dover, Mass.: Auburn House.

————. 1989. "Wages and Labor Supply in Rural India: The Role of Health, Nutrition and Seasonality." In David E. Sahn, ed., *Seasonal Variability in Third World Agriculture: The Consequences for Food Security*. Baltimore: Johns Hopkins University Press.

Behrman, Jere R., and Anil B. Deolalikar. 1987. "Will Developing Country Nutrition Improve with Income? A Case Study for Rural South India." *Journal of Political Economy* 95:492–507.

————. 1988a. "Impact of Macro Economic Adjustment on the Poor and on Social Sectors in Jamaica." Prepared for World Bank, Operations Evaluation Department. University of Pennsylvania, Department of Economics, Philadelphia. Processed.

————. 1988b. "Health and Nutrition." In Hollis B. Chenery and T. N. Srinivasan, eds., *Handbook of Development Economics*. Vol. 1. Amsterdam: North-Holland.

Behrman, Jere R., and Barbara L. Wolfe. 1987. "How Does Mother's Schooling Affect Family Health, Nutrition, Medical Care Usage, and Household Sanitation?" *Journal of Econometrics* 36:185–204.

Birdsall, Nancy, and Punham Chuhan. 1986. "Client Choice of Health Treatment in Rural Mali." World Bank, Population and Human Resources Department, Washington, D.C. Processed.

Birdsall, Nancy, François Orivel, Martha Ainsworth, and Punham Chuhan. 1983. "Three Studies on Cost Recovery in Social Sector

Projects." CPD Discussion Paper 1983-8. World Bank, Washington, D.C.

Boa, Jian Kang. 1987. "Results from the Hubei Province Household Survey." *Health Newspaper* 2507 (January 15). In Chinese.

Caldwell, John C. 1986. "Routes to Low Mortality in Poor Countries." *Population and Development Review* 12, no. 2 (June): 171–220.

Carrillo, E. R. 1986. "Health Care Facilities in Peru: A Health Sector Analysis of Peru." Technical Report. State University of New York at Stony Brook, Department of Economics. Processed.

Cline, W. R. 1983. *International Debt and the Stability of the World Economy.* Washington, D.C.: Institute for International Economics.

Cochrane, Susan H., D. J. O'Hara, and J. Leslie. 1980. *The Effects of Education on Health.* World Bank Staff Working Paper 405. Washington, D.C.

Colle, A. D., and M. Grossman. 1978. "Determinants of Pediatric Care Utilization." *Journal of Human Resources* 13 (supp.): 115–58.

Cornia, Giovanni A., Richard Jolly, and Frances Stewart. 1987. *Adjustment with a Human Face.* Oxford: Clarendon Press.

Cox, Karen M., and C. Geletkanycz. 1977. "The Health Situation in Peru." Department of Health, Education, and Welfare; Office of International Health; Department of Program Analysis; Washington, D.C.

Cretin, Shan, E. B. Keeler, A. P. Williams, and Y. Shi. 1988. "Factors Affecting Town-Countryside Differences in the Use of Health Services in Two Rural Counties in Sichuan." Rand Corporation, Santa Monica, Calif. Processed.

Davis, Karen, and L. B. Russel. 1972. "The Substitution of Hospital Outpatient Care for Inpatient Care." *Review of Economics and Statistics* 54:109–20.

Deaton, Angus, and John Muellbauer. 1980. *Economics and Consumer Behaviour.* Cambridge: Cambridge University Press.

De Ferranti, David. 1985. *Paying for Health Services in Developing Countries: An Overview.* World Bank Staff Working Paper 721. Washington, D.C.

Den Tuinder, Bastiaan A. 1978. *Ivory Coast, the Challenge of Success.* Baltimore: Johns Hopkins University Press.

Deolalikar, Anil B. 1988. "Nutrition and Labor Productivity in Agriculture: Estimates for Rural South India." *Review of Economics and Statistics* 70, no. 3 (August): 406–13.

Dor, Avi, and Jacques van der Gaag. 1988. *The Demand for Medical Care in Developing Countries: Quantity Rationing in Rural Côte d'Ivoire.* Living Standards Measurement Study Working Paper 35. Washington, D.C.: World Bank. Also forthcoming in K. Lee and A. Mills, eds., *Health Economic Research in Developing Countries.* New York: Oxford University Press.

Dor, Avi, Paul Gertler, and Jacques van der Gaag. 1987. "Non-Price Rationing and the Choice of Medical Care Providers in Rural Côte d'Ivoire." *Journal of Health Economics* 6:291–304.

Dunlop, David. 1987. "A Study of Health Financing: Issues and Options, Ethiopia." Sector Review. World Bank, Population and Human Resources Department, Washington, D.C. Processed.

Enyimayew, K. A. 1988. "Financing Drug Supplies of District Health Services in Ghana: The Ashanti-Akim Experience." Paper presented at the World Health Organization Workshop on Financing Drug Supplies, Harare, Zimbabwe, March.

Gereffi, G. 1988. "The Pharmaceuticals Market." In Dieter K. Zschock, ed., *Health Care in Peru: Resources and Policy.* Boulder, Colo.: Westview.

Gertler, Paul, L. Locay, and W. Sanderson. 1987. "Are User Fees Regressive? The Welfare Implications of Health Care Financing Proposals in Peru." *Journal of Econometrics* 36 (supp.): 67–88.

Gertler, Paul, and Jacques van der Gaag. 1988. *Measuring the Willingness to Pay for Social Services in Developing Countries.* Living Standards Measurement Study Working Paper 45. Washington, D.C.: World Bank.

Glewwe, Paul. 1988a. *The Distribution of Welfare in Côte d'Ivoire in 1985.* Living Standards Measurement Study Working Paper 29. Washington, D.C.: World Bank.

———. 1988b. *The Distribution of Welfare in Peru in 1985–86.* Living Standards Measurement Study Working Paper 42. Washington, D.C.: World Bank.

Goldman, Fred, and Michael Grossman. 1978. "The Demand for Pediatric Care: A Hedonic Appraisal." *Journal of Political Economy* 86:259–80.

Golladay, Frederick, and B. Liese. 1980. *Health Issues and Policies in the Developing Countries*. World Bank Staff Working Paper 412. Washington, D.C.

Heller, Peter. 1982. "A Model of the Demand for Medical and Health Services in Peninsular Malaysia." *Social Science and Medicine* 16:267–84.

Hensher, David A. 1986. "Sequential and Full Information Maximum Likelihood Estimation of a Nested Logit Model." *Review of Economics and Statistics* 68 (November): 657–67.

Hicks, Norman. 1980. *Economic Growth and Human Resources*. World Bank Staff Working Paper 408. Washington, D.C.

Holtmand, A. G., and E. O. Olsen. 1978. "The Demand for Dental Care: A Study of Consumption and Household Production." *Journal of Human Resources* 11:546–60.

Jimenez, Emmanuel. 1987. *Pricing Policy in the Social Sectors: Cost Recovery for Education and Health in Developing Countries*. Baltimore: Johns Hopkins University Press.

Kakwani, Nanak. 1988. "The Economic Crisis of the 1980s and Living Standards in Eighty Developing Countries." Centre for Applied Economic Research Paper 25. University of New South Wales, Australia.

Katz, Michael. 1987. "Pricing Publicly Supplied Goods and Services." In David Newbery and Nicholas Stern, eds., *The Theory of Taxation for Developing Countries*. New York: Oxford University Press.

Kravis, Irving B., Alan W. Heston, and Robert Summers. 1982. *World Product and Income: International Comparisons of Real Gross Product*. Baltimore: Johns Hopkins University Press.

Krueger, Anne O. 1968. "Factor Endowments and Per Capita Income Differences among Countries." *Economic Journal* 78:641–59.

Manning, Willard G., J. P. Newhouse, N. Daan, E. Keeler, B. Benjamin, A. Leibowitz, M. S. Marquis, and J. Zwanziger. 1987. *Health Insurance and the Demand for Medical Care*. Santa Monica, Calif.: Rand Corporation.

McFadden, Daniel Little. 1981. "Econometric Models of Probabilistic Choice." In Charles F. Manski and Daniel Little McFadden, eds., *Structural Analysis of Discrete Data with Econometric Applications*. Cambridge, Mass.: MIT Press.

Musgrove, Philip. 1978. *Consumer Behavior in Latin America: Income and Spending of Families in Ten Andean Cities*. Washington, D.C.: Brookings Institution.

―――. 1983. "Family Health Care Spending in Latin America." *Journal of Health Economics* 2:245–57.

Mwabu, Germano. 1986. "Health Care Decisions at the Household Level: Results of Health Survey in Kenya." *Social Science and Medicine* 22, no. 3: 313–19.

―――. 1988. "Conditional Logit Analysis of Household Choice of Medical Treatments in Rural Villages in Kenya." Kenyatta University, Department of Economics, Nairobi. Processed.

Newhouse, Joseph P. 1977. "Medical-Care Expenditure: A Cross-National Survey." *Journal of Human Resources* 12:115–25.

Newhouse, J. P., and C. E. Phelps. 1974. "Price and Income Elasticities from Medical Services." In Mark Perlman, ed., *The Economics of Health and Medical Care: Proceedings of a Conference Held by the International Economic Association at Tokyo*. New York: Wiley.

―――. 1976. "New Estimates of Price and Income Elasticities of Medical Services." In R. N. Rosett, ed., *The Role of Health Insurance in the Health Services Sector*. National Bureau of Economic Research Conference Series 27. New York.

Newman, John L. 1988. *Labor Market Activity in Côte d'Ivoire and Peru*. Living Standards Measurement Study Working Paper 36. Washington, D.C.: World Bank.

Newman, John, and Victor Lavy. 1988. "Labor Market and Adjustment during a Recession: The Micro and Macro Evidence." World Bank, Population and Human Resources Department, Washington, D.C. Processed.

Pan American Health Organization. 1982. *Health Conditions in the Americas*. Washington, D.C.

Phelps, C. E. 1975. "Effects of Insurance on Demand for Medical Care." In Ronald Anderson, Joanna Kravits, and Odin W. Anderson, eds., *Equity in Health Services*. Cambridge, Mass.: Ballinger.

―――. 1986. "Induced Demand: Can We Ever Know Its Extent?" *Journal of Health Economics* 5:355–65.

Phelps, C. E., and J. P. Newhouse. 1974. *Coinsurance and the Demand for Medical Services*. Publication R-964-2-OEO/NC. Santa Monica, Calif.: Rand Corporation.

Pollak, Robert A., and Michael L. Wachter. 1975. "The Relevance of the Household Production Function and Its Implications for the Allocation of Time." *Journal of Political Economy* 83:255–77.

Preston, Samuel A. 1980. "Causes and Consequences of Mortality in Less Developed Countries." In Richard A. Easterlin, ed., *Population and Economic Change in Developing Countries*. Chicago: University of Chicago Press.

Rao, Vijayendra. 1989. "Diet, Mortality, and Life Expectancy: A Cross-National Analysis." *Journal of Population Economics*.

Rosenzweig, Mark R., and T. Paul Schultz. 1982. "Child Mortality and Fertility in Colombia: Individual and Community Effects." *Health and Policy Education* 2, nos. 3–4: 305–48.

———. 1983. "Estimating a Household Production Function: Heterogeneity, the Demand for Health Inputs, and Their Effects on Birth Weight." *Journal of Political Economy* 91, no. 5: 723–46.

Rosenzweig, Mark R., and Kenneth I. Wolpin. 1986. "Evaluating the Effects of Optimally Distributed Public Programs: Child Health and Family Planning Interventions." *American Economic Review* 76, no. 3: 470–82.

Rosett, Richard N., and Lien-Fu Huang. 1973. "The Effect of Health Insurance on the Demand for Medical Care." *Journal of Political Economy* 81:281–305.

Sah, Raaj Kumar. 1987. "Queues, Rations, and Market: Comparisons of Outcomes for the Poor and the Rich." *American Economic Review* 77, no. 1 (March): 69–77.

Schwartz, J. B., J. S. Akin, and B. M. Popkin. 1988. "Price and Income Elasticities of Demand for Modern Health Care: The Case of Infant Delivery in the Philippines." *World Bank Economic Review* 2, no. 1: 49–76.

Small, K., and H. Rosen. 1981. "Applied Welfare Economics with Discrete Choice Models." *Econometrica* 1:105–30.

Strauss, John. 1986. "Does Better Nutrition Raise Farm Productivity?" *Journal of Political Economy* 94 (April): 297–320.

———. 1987. "Households, Communities and Preschool Children's Nutrition Outcomes: Evidence from Rural Côte d'Ivoire." Yale University, Economic Growth Center, New Haven, Conn. Processed.

———. 1988. *The Effects of Household and Community Characteristics on the Nutrition of Preschool Children: Evidence from Rural Côte d'Ivoire.* Living Standards Measurement Study Working Paper 40. Washington, D.C.: World Bank.

Suarez-Berenguela, Ruben M. 1988. *Financing the Health Sector in Peru.* Living Standards Measurement Study Working Paper 31. Washington, D.C.: World Bank.

Thomas, Duncan, John Strauss, and Maria Helena Henriques. 1987. "Child Survival, Nutritional Status and Household Characteristics: Evidence from Brazil." Yale University, Economic Growth Center, New Haven, Conn. Processed.

Train, Kenneth. 1986. *Qualitative Choice Analysis.* Cambridge, Mass.: MIT Press.

Van de Ven, Wynand P. M. M., and Jacques van der Gaag. 1982. "Health as an Unobservable: A MIMIC Model of Demand for Health Care." *Journal of Health Economics* 1:117–215.

Vogel, Ronald J. 1988. *Cost Recovery in the Health Care Sector.* World Bank Technical Paper 82. Washington, D.C.

Welch, W. P. 1985. "Health Care Utilization in HMO's: Results from Two National Samples." *Journal of Health Economics* 4:293–308.

Wheeler, David. 1980. *Human Resource Development and Economic Growth in Developing Countries: A Simultaneous Model.* World Bank Staff Working Paper 407. Washington, D.C.

Wolfe, Barbara L., and Jere R. Behrman. 1984. "Determinants of Women's Health Status and Health-Care Utilization in a Developing Country: A Latent Variable Approach." *Review of Economics and Statistics* 66, no. 4 (November): 696–703.

———. 1987. "Women's Schooling and Children's Health: Are the Effects Robust with Adult Sibling Control for the Women's Childhood Background?" *Journal of Health Economics* 6, no. 3 (September): 239–54.

World Bank. 1980. *World Development Report 1980.* New York: Oxford University Press.

————. 1986. "Social Indicators of Development." World Bank, Comparative Analysis and Data Division, Economic Analysis and Projections Department, Washington, D.C.

————. 1987. *Financing Health Services in Developing Countries*. World Bank Policy Study. Washington, D.C.

World Health Organization. 1987a. *Evaluation of the Strategy for Health for All by the Year 2000*. Geneva.

————. 1987b. *Economic Support for National Health for All Strategies*. Geneva.

Zschock, Dieter K. 1979. *Health Care Financing in Developing Countries*. Washington, D.C.: American Public Health Association.

————. 1980. "Health Care Financing in Central America and the Andean Region." *Latin America Research Review* 15, no. 3: 149–68.

————. 1983. "Medical Care under Social Insurance in Latin America: Review and Analysis." Agency for International Development, Bureau of Latin America and the Caribbean, Washington, D.C.

Index

Page numbers in italics indicate material in figures or in tables.

West Africa, health and health care
   in, 23–26. *See also* Côte d'Ivoire
Willingness to pay as against ability to pay, 56–59
World Bank, 2

The backlist of publications by the World Bank is shown in the annual *Index of Publications*, which is available from Publications Sales Unit, The World Bank, 1818 H Street, N.W., Washington, D.C. 20433, U.S.A., or from Publications, Banque mondiale, 66, avenue d'Iéna, 75116 Paris, France.